Practical Handbook of the
Temporal Bone and Middle Ear Cleft

Practical Handbook of the
Temporal Bone and Middle Ear Cleft

Neena H Bhalodiya MS (ENT) DLO
Professor and Head
Department of ENT
GMERS Medical College and Civil Hospital
Ahmedabad, Gujarat, India

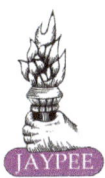

JAYPEE BROTHERS MEDICAL PUBLISHERS
The Health Sciences Publisher
New Delhi | London

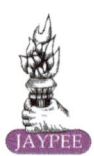 **Jaypee Brothers Medical Publishers (P) Ltd**

Headquarters

Jaypee Brothers Medical Publishers (P) Ltd
EMCA House, 23/23-B
Ansari Road, Daryaganj
New Delhi 110 002, India
Landline: +91-11-23272143, +91-11-23272703
+91-11-23282021, +91-11-23245672
Email: jaypee@jaypeebrothers.com

Corporate Office

Jaypee Brothers Medical Publishers (P) Ltd
4838/24, Ansari Road, Daryaganj
New Delhi 110 002, India
Phone: +91-11-43574357
Fax: +91-11-43574314
Email: jaypee@jaypeebrothers.com

Overseas Office

JP Medical Ltd
83 Victoria Street, London
SW1H 0HW (UK)
Phone: +44 20 3170 8910
Fax: +44 (0)20 3008 6180
Email: info@jpmedpub.com

Website: www.jaypeebrothers.com
Website: www.jaypeedigital.com

© 2023, Jaypee Brothers Medical Publishers

The views and opinions expressed in this book are solely those of the original contributor(s)/author(s) and do not necessarily represent those of editor(s) or publisher of the book.

All rights reserved. No part of this publication may be reproduced, stored or transmitted in any form or by any means, electronic, mechanical, photocopying, recording or otherwise, without the prior permission in writing of the publishers.

All brand names and product names used in this book are trade names, service marks, trademarks or registered trademarks of their respective owners. The publisher is not associated with any product or vendor mentioned in this book.

Medical knowledge and practice change constantly. This book is designed to provide accurate, authoritative information about the subject matter in question. However, readers are advised to check the most current information available on procedures included and check information from the manufacturer of each product to be administered, to verify the recommended dose, formula, method and duration of administration, adverse effects and contraindications. It is the responsibility of the practitioner to take all appropriate safety precautions. Neither the publisher nor the author(s)/editor(s) assume any liability for any injury and/or damage to persons or property arising from or related to use of material in this book.

This book is sold on the understanding that the publisher is not engaged in providing professional medical services. If such advice or services are required, the services of a competent medical professional should be sought.

Every effort has been made where necessary to contact holders of copyright to obtain permission to reproduce copyright material. If any have been inadvertently overlooked, the publisher will be pleased to make the necessary arrangements at the first opportunity.

Inquiries for bulk sales may be solicited at: jaypee@jaypeebrothers.com

Practical Handbook of the Temporal Bone and Middle Ear Cleft

First Edition: 2023

ISBN: 978-93-5465-884-6

Dedication

I want to dedicate this book to my Parents, Husband, and Mahek.

Preface

This book is aimed to exclusively cover the anatomy of the temporal bone and middle ear cleft. It explains embryology (development) and the anatomy of tympanic cavity, mastoid, eustachian tube, facial nerve, etc. along with its surgical implications. The content is both theoretical and practical. It will provide a basic idea regarding the dealing of these specific structures and the related complications during surgical procedures. I have tried to make explanations in-depth, but to the point. The book is written in a very simple and easy-to-understand language. It will be extremely important for budding ear, nose, and throat (ENT) surgeons and fellow ENTs.

Neena H Bhalodiya

Acknowledgments

- I want to thank everyone who helped me in making this book a reality.
- My teachers for all the learnings.
- A sincere gratitude of Dean, GMERS Medical College and Civil Hospital, Dr Nitin Vora and Medical Superintendent, GMERS Medical College and Civil Hospital, Dr Deepika Singhal. Special thanks to Dr Simple and Dr Chaitry.
- To all the present and past colleagues for your support and motivation.
- My dear residents who helped in writing this book—Swati, Kerul, Ravi, Parth Hingol, Nikki, Hardika, Parth Pomal, Pooja, Paridhi, Keval, Rinkal, Kushali, Kaivan, Nifla, and Dhawal.
- Dear Faculty of Audiology and SLP College, GMERS Medical College and Civil Hospital—Udit, Gunjan, Meenakshi, Mital, Jay, and Shubh.

Contents

1. The Temporal Bone 1
2. Middle Ear Cavity 11
3. Middle Ear Compartment 30
4. Facial Nerve 44
5. Eustachian Tube 56
6. Radiology of the Temporal Bone 61

Index *77*

Contents

CHAPTER 1

The Temporal Bone

INTRODUCTION

The temporal bone is complex bone situated at the sides and base of the skull and lateral to the temporal lobes of the cerebral cortex. It houses the structures of the ears, the facial nerve, and the internal carotid artery. The temporal bone consists of five bones: (1) The squamous, (2) the petrous, (3) the tympanic, (4) the mastoid, and (5) the styloid process **(Fig. 1)**.

DEVELOPMENT OF TEMPORAL BONE

It is the most complex anatomical structure, with multiple origins and development aspects.

Temporal bone develops from the eight ossification centers, one center for the squama, one for the tympanic part, four centers for petrous and mastoid bone, and two centers for the styloid process.

The temporal bone is an integral part of skull. The skull develops from the neurocranium, which surrounds the brain. The flat bones of the skull are derived from the intramembranous ossification which forms the vault. The base of skull (bones) is derived from the intracartilaginous ossification (squamous, occipital, sphenoid, ethmoid, petrous, and mastoid temporal). The viscerocranium which forms the facial bones is derived from the branchial arches **(Fig. 2)**.

The squamous bone forms the tegmen tympani, lateral wall of middle fossa, outer attic wall, and the lateral part of mastoid bone. The petrous bone (base) forms the medial wall of the entire middle ear cleft. The tympanic bone forms the external auditory meatus and the anterior and inferior (floor) walls of middle ear cavity **(Fig. 3A)**.

Styloid process, which is a slender, needle-like projection of the varying length (average 2–3 cm), projects from the inferior part of the petrous temporal bone. The squamous part is derived from the membranous neurocranium. In prenatal age, the squamous bone appears larger than the other bones. Apart from increase in size, the part of the squama which forms the fossa lies at the level of the zygomatic process, it thickens and contributes the middle cranial fossa. So, it becomes vertical and horizontal part.

The petromastoid part is developed from four centers. It appears as cartilaginous (otic) ear capsule. One center (prootic) appears near the arcuate prominence and extend to the apex of the bone. It forms the parts

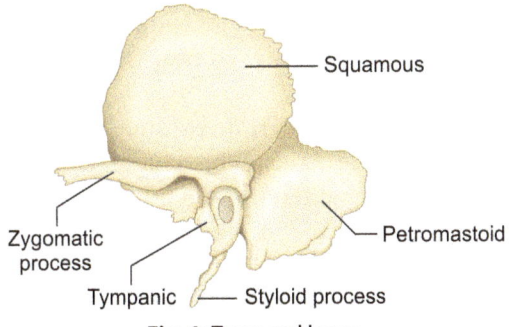

Fig. 1: Temporal bone.

2 The Temporal Bone

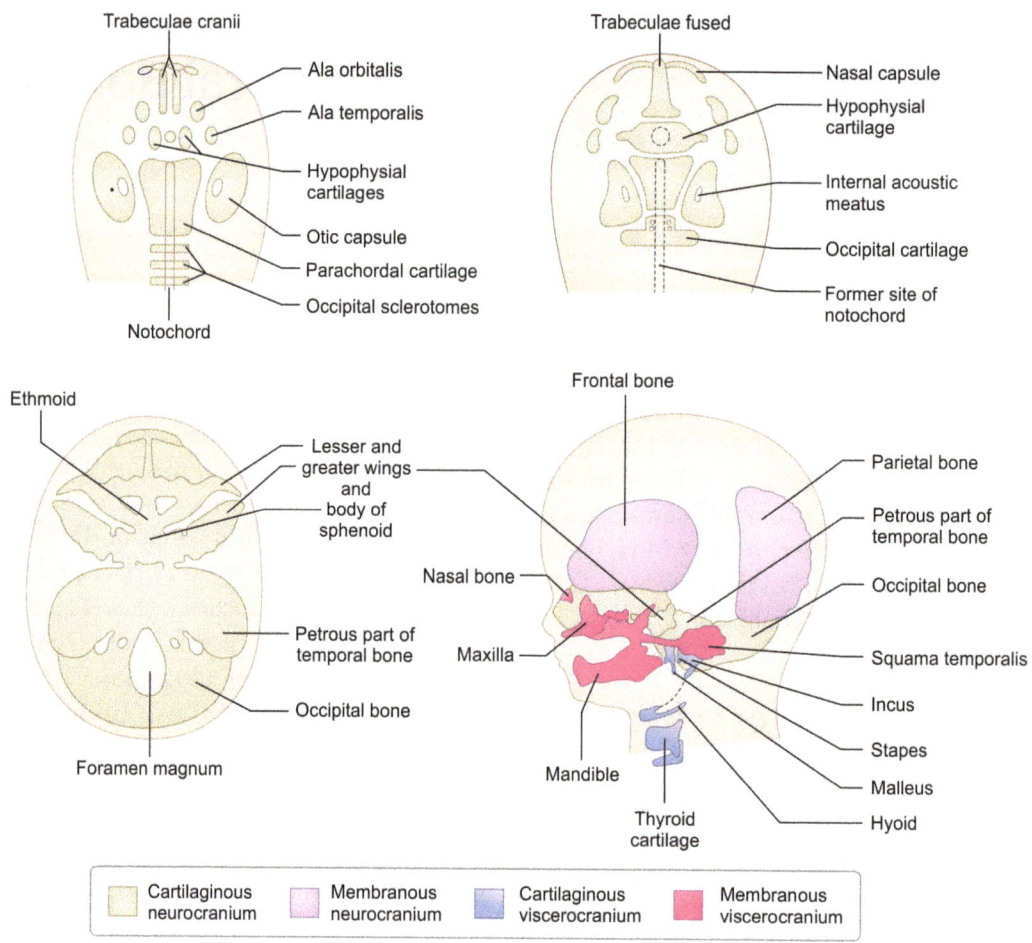

Fig. 2: Development of the human skull.

of cochlea, vestibule superior semicircular canal, and medial wall of tympanic cavity.

A second (opisthotic) appears at the promontory, it forms the floor of tympanic cavity and vestibule, surround the carotid canal and lower and lateral part of cochlea.

A third (pterotic) forms the roof of the tympanic cavity and antrum and the fourth (epiotic) appears near the posterior semicircular canal and extend to form the mastoid process **(Fig. 3B)**.

The tympanic ring is an incomplete ring in the concavity of which is groove tympanic sulcus for the attachment of the tympanic membrane. The styloid process is developed from the proximal part of the cartilage of the second branchial arch. The tympanic ring and the squama unite shortly before the birth. The petromastoid part and squama join during the first year. The styloid process unites till puberty.

The tympanic ring extends outward and backward to form the tympanic part. It extends more anteriorly and posteriorly. The meeting point of this outgrowth creates the foramen of Huschke. This foramen is usually closed about the fifth year of life but may persist throughout life.

The Temporal Bone

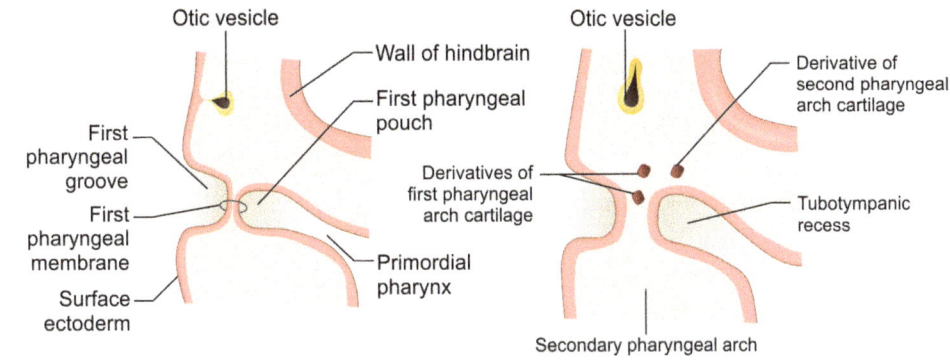

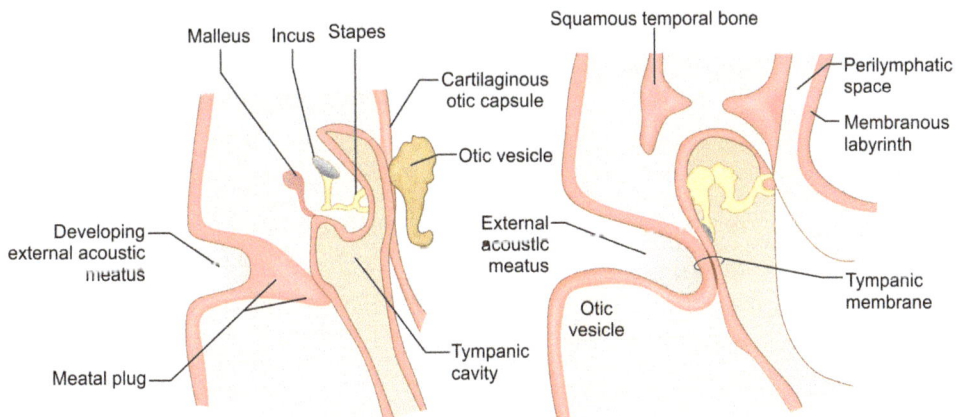

Fig. 3A: Development of ear.

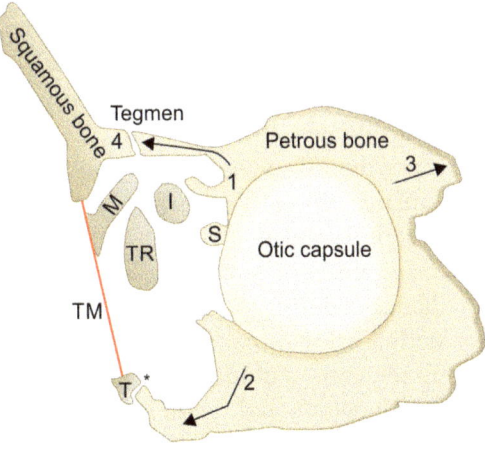

Fig. 3B: Development of structures from the otic capsule. Frontal plane. Cartilaginous projections emerge out from the otic capsule. (1) Lateral and superior projection grows from the otic capsule above the tubotympanic recess to form part of the tegmen tympani and walls of the ET. (2) Lateral and inferior projections form the jugular plate and the floor of the tympanic cavity. (3) Anteromedial part forms the petrous apex. The inferior wall of the middle ear is built up by the inferior plate of the petrous bone (2) which runs laterally to join the tympanic bone (T) *hypotympanic fissure. Tegmen tympani is formed by fusion of the tegmental process of the petrous bone (2) and the transverse process of squamous bone (4). (M: malleus; I: incus; S: stapes)

4 The Temporal Bone

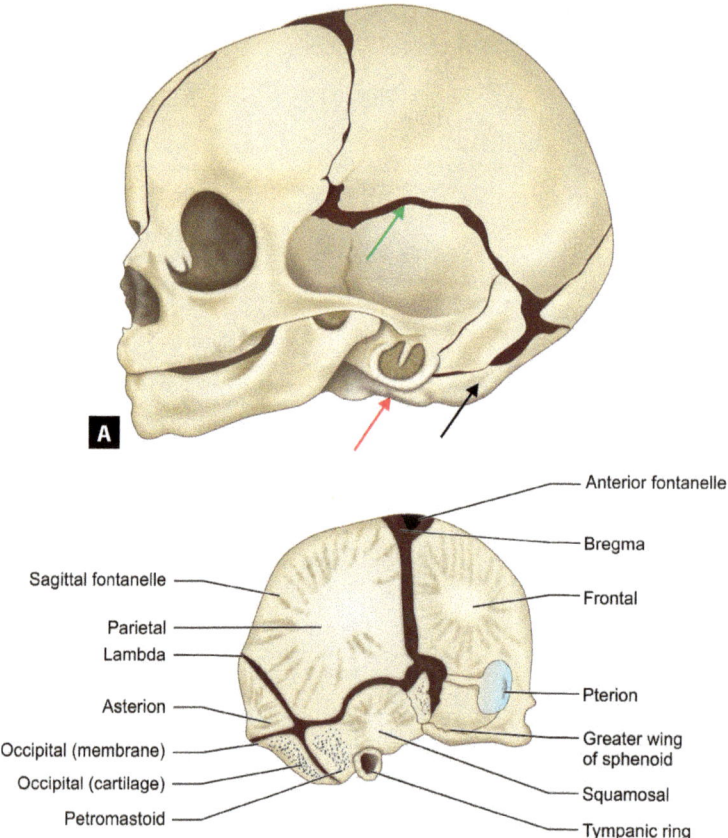

Figs. 4A and B: (A) Infant skull. [Flattened mastoid process (black arrow), stylomastoid foramen (red arrow, laterally displaced facial nerve), unfused sutures (green arrow)]; (B) A coronal section of the skull of 4-month-old fetus.
Source: Adapted from Shambaugh 6th edition.

The mastoid portion is flat at first, with stylomastoid foramen and rudimentary styloid just posterior to the tympanic ring. Within 1 year of age, the outer part of the mastoid grows anteroinferiorly to form mastoid process, with the styloid and the stylomastoid foramen shifting under the surface. The downward and forward growth of the mastoid process also pushes forward the tympanic part **(Figs. 4A and B)**.

- Normally, the foramen of Huschke disappears by the age of fifth year, but if persist, an evagination of skin of the external auditory canal (EAC) leads to the canal cholesteatoma.
- During development, the tympanic ring changes its orientation. At birth, the tympanic membrane is horizontal causing difficulty in exposure, then it becomes vertical.
- Facial nerve is superficial and may be damaged during forceps delivery.
- With a view of cochlear implantation, dimensions including tympanic cavity length, width, and depth of the mastoid should be adequately estimated. Cochlear wires should be placed with approximately

2.5 cm slacks to accommodate the anticipated growth.
- During developmental stage, fusion of the squamous and petrous part occurs. if failure of fusion persists between squamous and petrous part of mastoid, it forms the Korner's septum. On the outer surface, external petromastoid suture is visualized.

SURFACE ANATOMY OF THE TEMPORAL BONE

The temporal bone is fused to the sphenoid, parietal, occipital, and zygomatic bones and contributes to the cranial, skull base, and facial structures.

The temporal bone has a pyramidal shape, the sides of which forms the middle fossa floor (superior face), the anterior limit of the posterior cranial fossa (posterior face), muscle attachment of the neck and infratemporal fossa (anterior-inferior face), and the muscular-cutaneous-covered side of the head (lateral) which forms the base of the pyramid.

The temporal bone paired, symmetrical bone, derived from the fusion of the petrous, the squamous, the tympanic, and styloid bone.

Petrous Bone

The Greek word "Petra" means solid, hard bone. It has shape of pyramid whose base is united with mastoid laterally; the apex is oriented anteromedially between the occipital and sphenoid bone. The jugular foramen is formed at the junction between the petrous and occipital bone (at the clivus). This foramen is partitioned by the jugular spine into the anterior pars venosa and posterior pars nervosa.

The petrous bone **(Fig. 5)** contains important structures: Semi-circular canal,

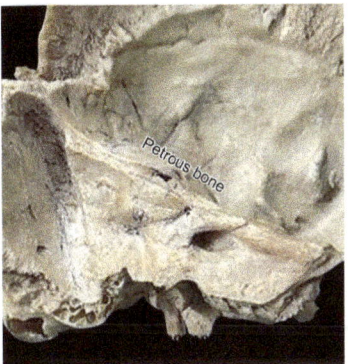

Fig. 5: Petrous part of the temporal bone.

cochlea, vestibule (labyrinth), the facial nerve, and internal carotid artery. It forms the medial wall of the tympanic cavity, aditus ad antrum, and the mastoid.

The petrous bone articulates with the tympanic, mastoid, and squamous bone. It leads to the formation of intrinsic fissures:

Petrosquamous Fissures

This fissure connects the petrous and squamous bone.
- *External petrosquamous fissure:* It appears on the outer lateral surface of mastoid process.
- *Internal petrosquamous fissure:* It is present in the roof the tympanic cavity (tegmen tympani) and joins its parts.

Petrotympanic Fissures (Glassarian Fissures) (Fig. 6)

It is situated between the mandibular fossa and the medial aspect of the tympanic bone. It transmits three structures: The chorda tympani nerve, the anterior tympanic artery, and the anterior malleal ligament.

The petrous pyramid has an anterior surface, posterior surface, and the inferior surface.

The anterior surface forms the postero-medial surface of the middle fossa floor.

The Temporal Bone

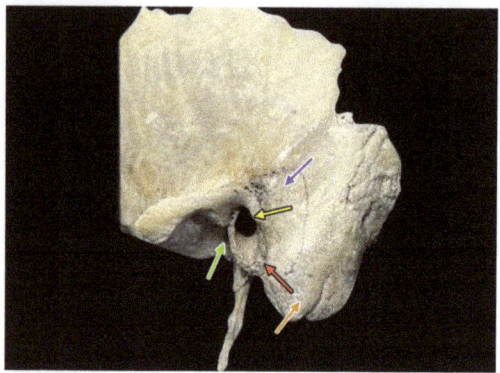

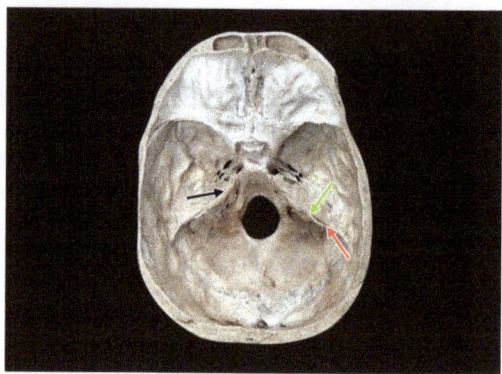

Fig. 6: Petrotympanic fissure in the temporal bone. [Mastoid tip (orange arrow); tympanomastoid fissure (red arrow); petrotympanic fissure (green arrow); tympanosquamous suture (purple arrow); spine of Henle (yellow arrow)].

Fig. 8: Superior surface of temporal bone with posterior face of petrous bone. [Petrous apex (black arrow); Groove for superior petrosal sinus (red arrow); arcuate eminence (green arrow)].

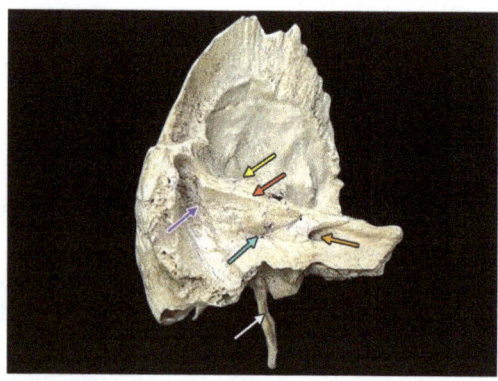

Fig. 7: Anterior surface of petrous bone with landmarks. [Arcuate eminence (yellow arrow); vestibular duct opening (purple arrow); internal auditory meatus (orange arrow); Groove for superior petrosal sinus (red arrow); styloid process (white arrow)].

Prominent surface features include medially, arcuate eminence (by prominence of superior semi-circular canal) and sulcus of the superior petrosal sinus **(Fig. 7)**. Junction of petrous bone with the greater wing of sphenoid bone, the musculoskeletal canal containing more superficial semi canal of the tensor tympani and a deeper semi canal of the auditory tube. At the apex, smooth depression occupied by the trigeminal ganglion, just posterior to sulci of greater and lesser petrosal nerves. Parallel to the sphenoid suture line. The roof of the middle ear and mastoid extends lateral to the arcuate eminence.

The posterior surface of the petrous bone is oriented in the vertical plane forming the anterior bony limit of the posterior fossa. This surface is framed by the sigmoid sinus, the superior and inferior petrosal sinuses. At the center of the surface, porus acoustics or internal auditory meatus is visualized. It has two ends, fundus (lateral) end and porous (medial) end **(Fig. 8)**.

The subarcuate artery emerges from a fossa which is located superior and lateral to the acoustic meatus (subarcuate fossa), whereas the endolymphatic sac and duct occupy the depression and opening located inferolaterally known as the operculum.

The inferior surface of temporal bone is irregular due to attachments of the multiple muscles. Medial to the mastoid tip, the posterior belly of digastric muscle is inserted in a sulcus which terminates anteriorly at the stylomastoid foramen. The styloid process is

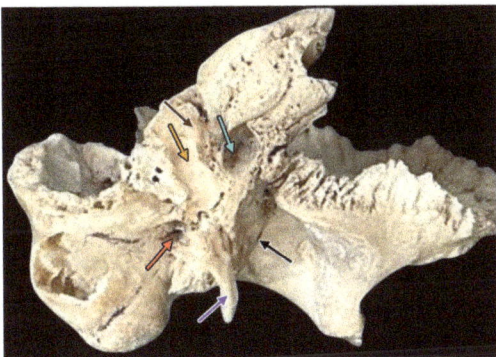

Fig. 9: Inferior surface of the temporal bone. [Stylomastoid foramen (red arrow); tympanosquamous fissure (black arrow); styloid process (purple arrow); carotid canal (blue arrow); Jugular fossa (orange arrow); cochlear aqueduct (brown arrow)].

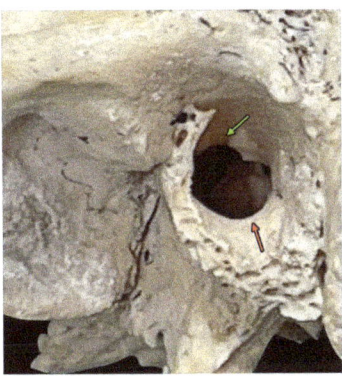

Fig. 10: Tympanic part of the temporal bone. [Scutum (green arrow); tympanic ring (red arrow)].

located anteriorly to this process and both are located at the anterior limit in line with the digastric groove. Medial and parallel to the digastric groove is a sulcus for the occipital artery **(Fig. 9)**.

Jugular foramen lies directly under the middle ear space. The jugular bulb is located in the jugular fossa, lateral to the jugular foramen. The inferior foramen of the carotid canal lies anterior to the jugular bulb depression and it is separated by a wedge-shaped bone called keel. The tympanic canaliculus penetrates this keel to transmit sensory and preganglionic parasympathetic fibers of the inferior ganglion of the glossopharyngeal nerve into the middle ear as Jacobson's nerve. The jugular spine which divides the jugular fossa into the anterior and posterior compartment, the external aperture of the cochlear aqueduct lies anterior and medial to this jugular spine, the cochlear aqueduct eventually opens into the Scala tympani at the cochlear base. In the translabyrinthine approach to the internal auditory canal (IAC), the cochlear aqueduct is the inferior limit of dissection used to avoid injury to lower cranial nerves.

The Tympanic Bone (Fig. 10)

It is a C-shaped plate of bone situated between the glenoid fossa anteriorly and the mastoid process posteriorly. It forms the anterior wall, floor, part of the posterior wall, and the roof of the bony EAC and anterior wall and floor of the middle ear cavity. The anterior edge of this open ring forms the tympanosquamous suture line within the EAC, and the petrotympanic suture line within the middle ear, through which the chorda tympani exist middle ear.

The posterior edge of the tympanic ring forms the tympanomastoid suture line which curves from the posterior EAC inferiorly up to the stylomastoid foramen serving as landmark for the facial nerve as it exits the temporal bone.

Vaginal process of the tympanic bone is plate which surrounds the styloid process and fuse with the petrous bone near the carotid canal. The tympanic ring is deficient superiorly near the attachment of the squamous bone known as the "Notch of Rivinus."

The Squamous Part (Fig. 11)

It forms the lateral wall of the middle fossa. It consists of outer and inner cortical plates

The Temporal Bone

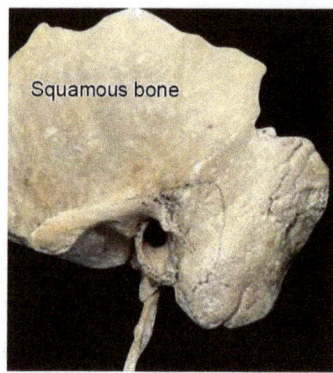

Fig. 11: Squamous part of the temporal bone.

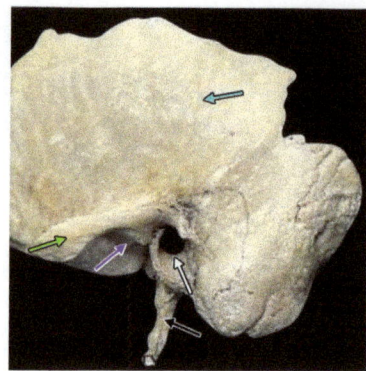

Fig. 12: Mastoid bone forming the lateral surface of the temporal bone. [External auditory meatus (white arrow); mandibular fossa (purple arrow); zygomatic process (green arrow); styloid process (black arrow); Groove for middle temporal artery (blue arrow)].

with anterior extension known as the zygomatic process which forms the bony roof of the glenoid fossa. A horizontal ridge, the temporal line, is formed along the most inferior insertion of the temporalis muscle which is aligned with the zygomatic process. The temporal line provides a first approximation for the location of the middle fossa floor which on average is positioned ~4.7 mm inferiorly.

The squamous portion has two parts—(1) vertical and (2) horizontal. The vertical squama part forms the lateral wall of middle cranial fossa while the horizontal part forms part of roof of middle ear cavity and scutum (outer attic wall).

The Mastoid Bone (Fig. 12)

It is a bulbous bony structure shaped by expansion of air-filled space within and constant pull of the mastoid muscle (sternocleidomastoid and digastric) elongates the mastoid inferiorly and anteriorly form mastoid tip (process). The mastoid cortex is perforated by the emissary vessels which drain from the central air cell (antrum) and forming triangular McEwan's triangle and depressed cribriform area at the junction of the mastoid with the tympanic bone. The foramen of emissary vein is visualized near the posterior limit of the outer cortex and communicates with the sigmoid sinus.

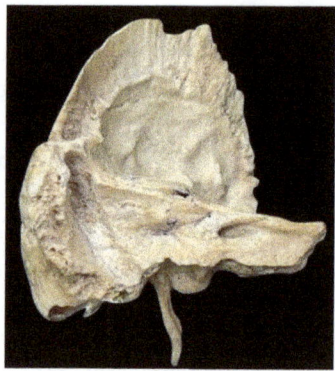

Fig. 13: The styloid bone.

The Styloid Process (Fig. 13)

It is pointed, slender needle-like projection between the external and internal carotid arteries.

Styloid apparatus is formed by the attachment of three muscles and two ligaments. It is found within the parapharyngeal space. The stylohyoid innervated by the facial nerve

(7th), the stylopharyngeus muscle innervated by the glossopharyngeal nerve (9th), and a styloglossus innervated by the hypoglossal nerve (12th).

Two ligaments, the stylomandibular ligament and the stylohyoid ligament, contribute to the styloid apparatus.

- Developmental arrest of the temporal bone at different stages gives rise to variety of congenital malformations, such as atresia of external ear, ossicle, and labyrinthine anomalies.
- In case of deaf and mute patients, we should read the radiography of the temporal bone properly to find out various congenital anomalies of labyrinthine and associated malformations of facial nerve, middle ear, and external ear.
- Presence of Korner's septum may give a false apprehension of entry into mastoid antrum.
- MacEwen triangle is also called as triangle of attack and is a landmark for mastoid antrum.
- Subarcuate fossa and petromastoid cell which open into mastoid antrum may give rise to intracranial infections.
- Fissures in the temporal bone may resemble fracture line and may result in faulty diagnosis.
- In middle cranial fossa approach for cerebellopontine (CP) angle tumor, one must identify the greater superficial petrosal nerve and arcuate eminence to know the location of IAC.
- Computed tomography scan of the temporal bone may show erosion of keel (caroticojugular crest) in cases of glomus jugulare.
- For a translabyrinthine approach, the inferior limit is the cochlear aqueduct to prevent injury to the lower cranial nerves.
- *For cochlear implant:* Width of internal auditory meatus gives idea about the presence of cochlear nerves and a deficient cribriform area gives rise to perilymphatic gusher.

BIBLIOGRAPHY

1. Anson BJ, Bast TH, Richamy SF. The fetal and early postnatal development of the tympanic ring and related structures in man. Ann Otol Rhinol Laryngol. 1955;64(3):802-22.
2. Ars B, Ars-Piret N. Mouvements embryogéniques de l'anneau tympanique. In: Martin H (Ed). Comptes rendus du Congrès de la Société Française d'ORL. Paris: Arnette; 1981. pp. 117-9.
3. Ars B, Decraemer W, Marquet J, Ars-Piret N. Sulcustympanicus. In: Comptes-rendusduCongrès de la Société Française d'ORL. Paris: Arnette; 1980. pp. 401 68.
4. Ars B. Le foramen de Huschke. Acta Otorhinolaryngol Belg. 1988;42:654-8.
5. Ars B. La partie tympanale de l'os temporal. Cahiers ORL. 1983;18:435-523.
6. Ars B. Pars Tympanica Ossis Temporalis. Academicalthesis, thèse d'agrégation de l'Enseignement supérieur. Belgium: University of Antwerp; 1982.
7. Clerc P, Batisse R. [Approach to the intrapetrosal organs by the endocranial route; graft of the facial nerve]. Ann Otolaryngol. 1954;71(1):20-38.
8. Dobozi M. Surgical anatomy of the geniculate ganglion. Acta Otolaryngol. 1975; 80(1-2):116-9.
9. Eby TL, Nadol JB. Postnatal growth of the human temporal bone. Implications for cochlear implants in children. Ann Otol Rhinol Laryngol. 1986;95(4 Pt 1):356-64.
10. Gulya AJ. Developmental anatomy of the temporal bone and skull base. In: Glasscock ME, Gulya AJ (Eds). Glasscock Shambaugh Surgery of the Ear, 5th edition. Hamilton: BC Decker Inc; 2003. pp. 4-7.
11. Gözil R, Yener N, Calgüner E, Araç M, Tunç E, Bahcelioğlu M. Morphological characteristics of styloid process evaluated

by computerized axial tomography. Ann Anat. 2001;183(6):527-35.
12. Jung T, Tschernitschek H, Hippen H, Schneider B, Borchers L. Elongated styloid process: when is it really elongated? Dentomaxillofac Radiol. 2004;33(2):119-24.
13. Kartush JM, Kemink JL, Graham MD. The arcuate eminence. Topographic orientation in middle cranial fossa surgery. Ann Otol Rhinol Laryngol. 1985;94(1 Pt 1):25-8.
14. Kolagi S, Herur A, Ugale M, Manjula R, Mutalik A. Suboccipital retrosigmoid surgical approach for internal auditory canal: a morphometric anatomical study on dry human temporal bones. Indian J Otolaryngol Head Neck Surg. 2010;62(4):372-5.
15. Mallo M, Gridley T. Development of the mammalian ear: coordinate regulation of formation of the tympanic ring and the external acoustic meatus. Development. 1996;122(1):173-9.
16. Moffat DA, Ramsden RT, Shaw HJ. The styloid process syndrome: aetiological factors and surgical management. J Laryngol Otol. 1977;91(4):279-94.
17. Rhoton Jr AL, Pulec JL, Hall GM, Boyd Jr AS. Absence of bone over the geniculate ganglion. J Neurosurg. 1968;28(1):48-53.
18. Roche PH, Mercier P, Sameshima T, Fournier HD. Surgical anatomy of the jugular foramen. Adv Tech Stand Neurosurg. 2008;33:233-63.
19. Simms DL, Neely JG. Growth of the lateral surface of the temporal bone in children. Laryngoscope. 1989;99(8 Pt 1):795-9.
20. Tardivet L. Anatomie Chirurgicale du nerf facial intra-petreux, Thèse Med. France: Aix Marseille University; 2003.
21. Yamada G, Mansouri A, Torres M, Stuart ET, Blum M, Schultz M, et al. Targeted mutation of the murine goosecoid gene results in craniofacial defects and neonatal death. Development. 1995;121(9):2917-22.

CHAPTER 2

Middle Ear Cavity

DEVELOPMENT OF THE EAR

The temporal bone and the structures of the ear develop from the neurocranium and the brachial arches.

DEVELOPMENT OF THE EXTERNAL EAR

At 4 weeks of intrauterine life, tissue condensation of the first brachial (mandibular) and second (hyoid) arch appears at the distal portion of the first brachial groove.

This tissue condensation develops into six ridges "The hillock of His". These hillocks fuse to form two folds which again fuse superiorly and form the pinna. The entire pinna, except tragus, arises from the second brachial arch and anterior part of the external auditory canal (EAC) arises from the first pharyngeal arch. It reaches to adult configuration at fifth month, independent of progress in middle and inner ears.

DEVELOPMENT OF TYMPANOMASTOID COMPARTMENT AND THE AUDITORY TUBE

This includes the development of the tympanic ring, the tympanic membrane, middle ear cavity with contents, and Eustachian tube.

External auditory canal develops from the dorsal part of the first brachial groove, while outpouching of the first brachial pouch gives rise to tubotympanic recess (**Flowchart 1**) at third week of intrauterine life. The ectoderm of the first pharyngeal groove abuts on the endoderm of the tubotympanic recess. At sixth week, a mesodermal ingrowth breaks this.

A cord of epithelial cells, at the depth of primary EAC, grows medially into mesenchyme and develops into solid-meatal plate. The mesenchyme adjacent to the meatal plate gives rise to the lamina propria of the tympanic membrane and at 9 weeks, it is surrounded by four ossification centers of tympanic ring.

The components of the tympanic ring fuses by 10th week, except superiorly, where a defect remains as the notch of Rivinus (**Fig. 1**). At the beginning of the 4th month, the squama projects posterior to the tympanic ring forming the lateral part of mastoid, roof of the EAC. After the 8th month, the tympanic ring starts to fuse with the otic capsule and the growth continues after birth. The styloid process appears after birth from the Reichert's cartilage.

Due to the abnormal development of the first and second branchial arches; microtia, anotia, or abnormal position of pinna occurs. External ear canal stenosis or atresia arise as noncanalization of 1st branchial groove. Deformity of middle ear or inner ear depends upon the time when development is affected.

At the 3rd week, an outpouching of the first branchial pouch known as tubotympanic

12 Middle Ear Cavity

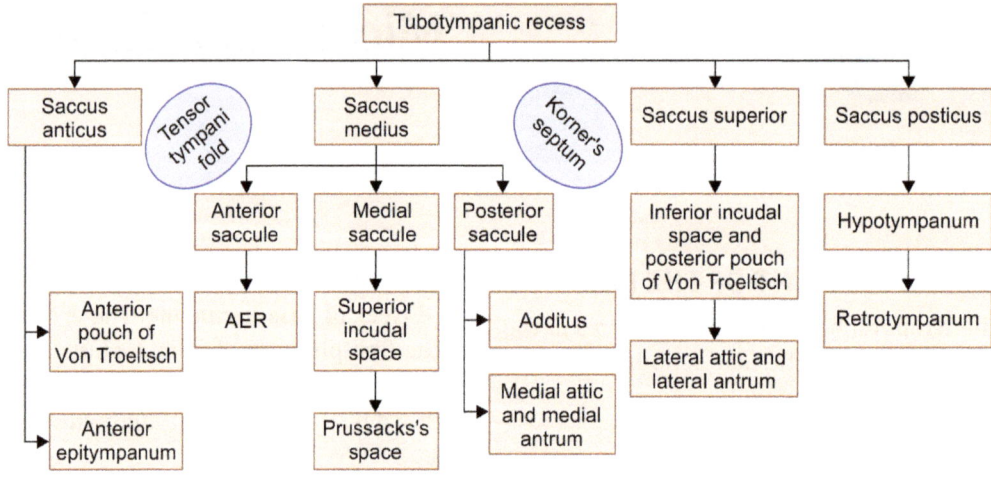

Flowchart 1: The embryology of the middle ear spaces from tubotympanic recess.

(AER: anterior epitympanic recess)

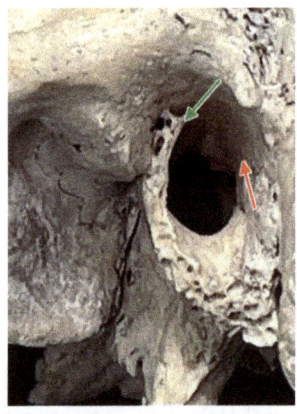

Fig. 1: Anterior and posterior tympanic spines in the tympanic bone showing the anterior and posterior limits of Notch of Rivinus. [Anterior tympanic spine (green arrow); posterior tympanic spine (red arrow)].

recess eventually becomes the Eustachian tube and tympanic cavity. At 7th week, because of simultaneous growth of the second brachial arch, tubotympanic recess constricts at midpoint.

So primordial tympanic cavity lies laterally, while primordial Eustachian tube lies medially. The Eustachian tube develops very remarkably, it lengthens and becomes narrow with mesodermal development and fibrocartilaginous tube is established.

The terminal end of the first pharyngeal (endothelial) pouch develops into four sacci (anticus, posticus, superior, and medial) which expand and pneumatize the tympanic cavity **(Fig. 2)**.

Saccus anticus is the smallest sacci and forms anterior epitympanic recess and anterior pouch of Von Troeltsch. Mucosal fold develops ossicles by this sacci, which lines the tympanomastoid compartment. The part where these mucosal lining join transmits the blood vessels.

DEVELOPMENT OF THE OSSICULAR CHAIN

The pharyngeal arches have three layers: Ectoderm, mesoderm, and endoderm. Ectodermal cleft gives rise to the external auditory meatus and outer epithelial layer of the tympanic membrane with unique property of skin migration laterally. Endodermal pouch gives rise to tubotympanic recess. Mesoderm of this brachial arches forms the

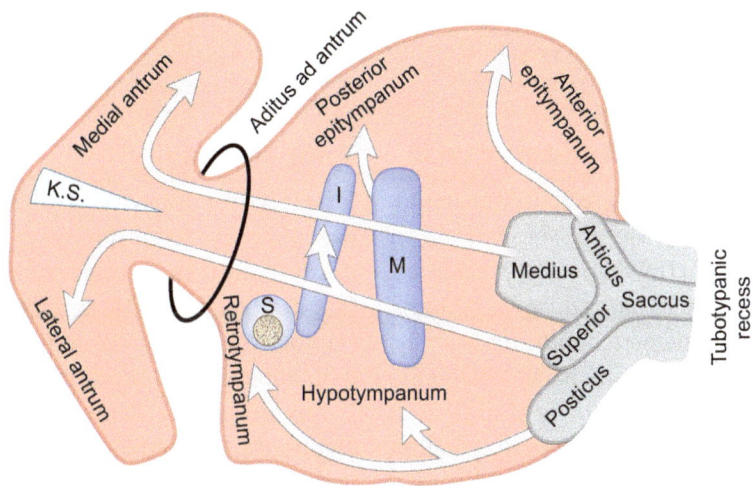

Fig. 2: The embryology of the middle ear spaces. (I: incus; M: malleus; S: stapes; K.S.: Korner's septum)

content of tympanic cavity (ossicles, muscles, and nerves and vessels).

Approximately at 4 weeks, ossicles appear as interbrachial bridge which is mesenchymal bridge between first and second brachial arch, differentiation of it forms primordial malleus and incus. The stapes blastema arises from the 2nd branchial arch (annular ligament and medial side of footplate derived from otic capsule).

After 11 weeks, cartilaginous ossicles develop, the anterior process of malleus develops as membranous ossification. The stapedial artery encircles the stapes blastema. As stapedial artery disappears, it leaves behind an empty obturator foramen.

By 15th week, the ossicles attain adult size and then ossification starts. First in the incus, followed by malleus and stapes sequentially. There is simultaneous development of the tensor tympani and stapedius from the mesenchyme of these arches. Adult size configuration of ossicles reached by 20 weeks and stapes reduce to it normal size up to 32 weeks.

DEVELOPMENT OF THE MASTOID

Outer (lateral) part of the mastoid is derived from the squamous bone and medial part of the mastoid, from the petrous bone. Pneumatization of mastoid appears at 33 weeks, then it proceeds surrounding air cells tracts. Pneumatization depends upon hereditary factors, environment, nutrition, bacterial infection, and ventilation by the auditory tube.

Antrum achieves approximately adult size at the time of birth, and it proceeds up to 1 year with mesenchymal resolution. Mastoid continues to grow very slowly up to puberty.

ANATOMY

The tympanomastoid compartment includes tympanic cavity, mastoid air cell system, connecting auditory tube as well as EAC.

Middle ear cleft is sagittally oriented air-containing space from the Eustachian tube to the mastoid antrum. External ear, middle ear, and inner ear have potential for the transmission of sound and balance (axis parallel to petrous ridge). Tympanic cavity lies at the crossing of both the axis.

Pinna and External Auditory Canal

The pinna focuses and localizes the sound. The shape of pinna varies. The contour of pinna is determined by yellow elastic cartilage. Attachment of skin to the cartilage is different (tightly attach to the perichondrium laterally, while loose attachment medially). The pinna skin has hairs and sebaceous glands. It is continuous with cartilage of canal as well as tympanic bone. The postauricular nerve, branch of facial nerve, supplies the muscle.

External Auditory Meatus

Lateral cartilaginous (1/3rd) and medial bony meatus (2/3rd). There is deficient area of cartilage known as incisura terminalis. This gap is utilized in the endaural incision. The narrowest part of the canal lies just medial to junction of bony and cartilaginous part known as isthmus. Skin of the bony external canal is very thin (absence of hairs), only 0.2 mm in thickness, it requires meticulous shaped dissection between anterosuperior (tympanosquamous suture) and posteroinferior (tympanomastoid suture). The pinna and EAC get innervation by facial nerve, auriculotemporal nerve (trigeminal nerve), greater auricular and lesser occipital nerve (c2, c3 connection), and auricular branch of vagus nerve.
- For local anesthesia, infiltration is done in a four quadrant (at 2, 4, 8, 10 o'clock)
- *Vascular strips:* Tympanosquamous and tympanomastoid suture defines the sites for incisions.
- Inflammatory condition of the external ear is painful due to its adherence to the cartilage.
- Perichondrium of the pinna starts to necrose as blood supply is affected and it gets deformity after 3 days.

Tympanic Cavity

It is air-filled cavity connecting to the nasopharynx by the auditory tube and to the mastoid antrum through aditus ad antrum (sagittally oriented). It is air containing (around 2cc) and it transmits the sound from the tympanic membrane to the oval window. Tympanic cavity containing an ossicular chain and ligaments which connect wall of tympanic cavity.

Tympanic cavity considered as box with roof (tegmen tympani), a floor (bone separating jugular bulb), and four walls (anterior, posterior, medial, and lateral). Medial wall and lateral wall have convexity, so it is constricted in the middle (varying depth of the cavity) **(Fig. 3)**.

Tympanic cavity is developed from the tubotympanic recess. Otic capsule extends the cartilaginous rim laterally toward the tubotympanic recess superiorly, inferiorly, anteriorly, and posteriorly. This way petrous bone forms medial wall of the middle ear cleft. Lateral and anterior wall is formed by the tympanic bone. Posterior wall is formed by the Reichert' cartilage.

Roof of the Tympanic Cavity (Tegmen Tympani) (Figs. 4A and B)

The tegmen plate is a bony plate which separates the middle ear cleft and middle cranial fossa. Tegmen plate above the middle ear cavity is known as tegmen tympani, while above the mastoid antrum and Eustachian tube is the tegmen antri and tegmen tubari, respectively.

Tegmen is formed by the petrous bone and the squamous bone. It is not horizontal.

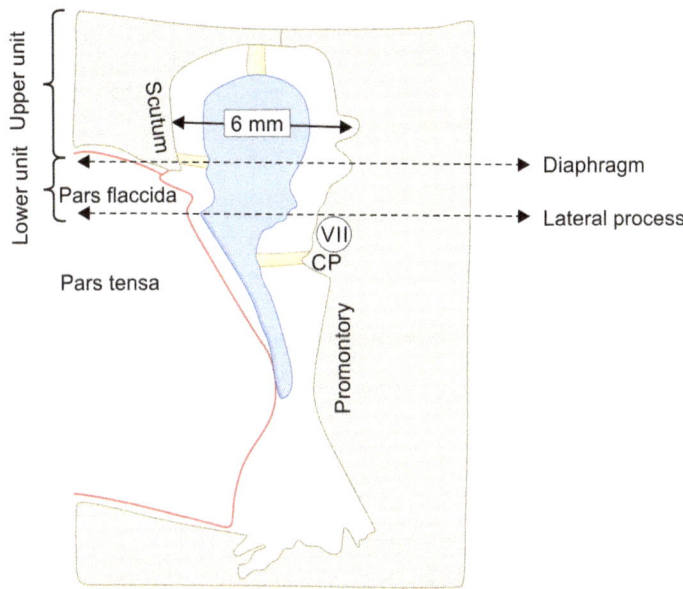

Fig. 3: Middle ear cavity with its dimensions. (Upper unit and lower unit of the attic; VII: facial nerve; CP: cochleariform process)

Plate of bone in tympani, tegmental process of the petrous bone covers the roof of anterior attic, while posterior part of the attic and the antrum are covered by the horizontal process of squamous bone and the tegmental process of petrous bone. The entire tegmen is formed with strength of junction of two bones.

This plate is not horizontal, there are two slopes: (1) From lateral to medial side. It slopes inferiorly from medial to lateral (high at the level of superior semicircular canal). (2) From posterior to anterior: As from mastoid antrum to the zygomatic area, it slopes down gradually placing the tegmen higher anteriorly.

Subarachnoid space surrounding the facial nerve extends up to the geniculate ganglion and very rarely, it can create cerebrospinal fluid (CSF) fistula in the middle ear through the tegmen tympani.

Cog is coronally oriented bony plate of the tegmen tympani toward the cochleariformis process and anterior to the head of malleus.

The cog is located superiorly to the facial nerve with its tip pointing to it. The cog is one of the landmarks for the tympani segment of facial nerve.

In tympanomastoid surgeries, preservation of the tegmen tympani is very important. It is not horizontal plate.

Floor of the Tympanic Cavity

It is irregularly contoured floor which separates the mesotympanum and the hypotympanum and features the jugular bulb and root of styloid process posteriorly and internal carotid artery (ICA) anteriorly **(Fig. 5)**.

The hypotympanum develops between 22 and 32 weeks as fusion of three bones: (1) Tympanic bone (membranous bone), (2) Canalicular otic capsule (endochondral bone), and (3) a petrosal bone (periosteal bone). These structures are thought to predispose this area for the abnormal development such as dehiscent jugular bulb. Incomplete fusion leads to formation

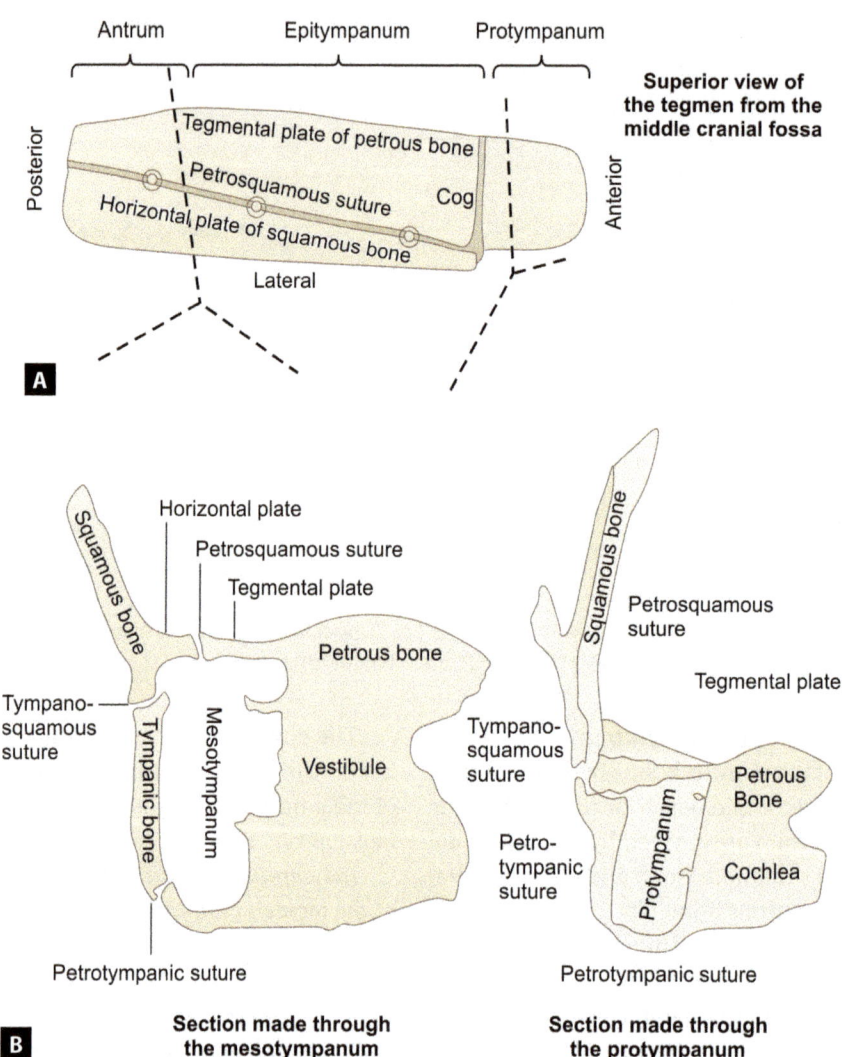

Figs. 4A and B: Superior wall of the middle ear cavity.

of the hypotympanic fissure which leads to inferior canaliculi through which branch of the inferior tympanic artery and Jacobson nerve enter tympanic cavity. The jugular bulb lies in the floor of the tympanic cavity which connects the lateral sinus to internal jugular vein. The jugular bulb is situated medial to the vertical segment of facial nerve and inferior to the posterior semicircular canal. The lower cranial nerve (9th, 10th, and 11th) exits the skull through jugular foramen. Bony or fibrous compartmentalization of foramen leads to anteromedial compartment with glossopharyngeal nerve, whereas cranial nerve X and XI and the jugular bulb located posterolaterally.

The inferior petrosal sinus through its multiple opening in the anterior aspect of jugular bulb, closely related to the glossopharyngeal nerve.

- The jugular foramen is of particular importance in skull base surgery.

Middle Ear Cavity

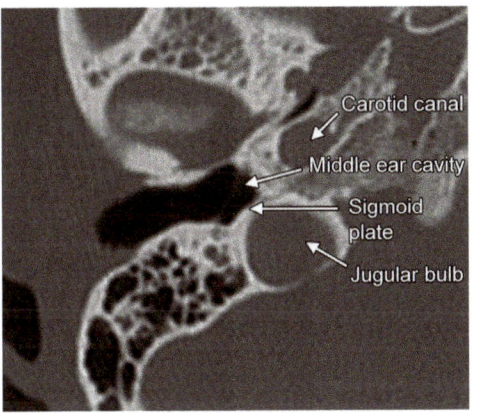

Fig. 5: Computed tomography (CT) scan axial cut showing floor of tympanic cavity with jugular bulb and internal carotid artery.

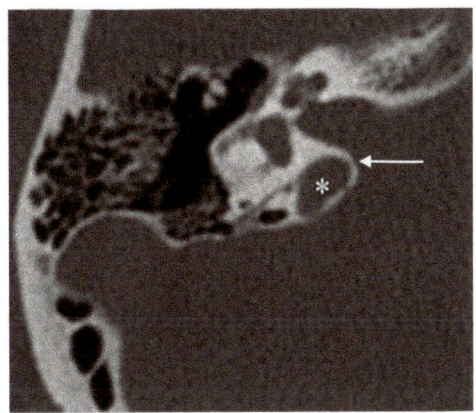

Fig. 6: Computed tomography (CT) scan axial cut showing high riding jugular bulb. [High riding jugular bulb (asterix)].

- *Retrofacial approach:* Hypotympanic space can be approached medial to the mastoid segment of the facial nerve and inferior to the posterior semicircular canal. High and lateral jugular bulb make this approach difficult.
- *High jugular bulb:* Jugular bulb can rise up to the petrous ridge **(Fig. 6)**.
- *Dehiscent jugular bulb:* If covering bony plate is absent make the exposed jugular bulb in the middle ear cavity **(Fig. 7)**.
- In translabyrinthine approach for cerebellopontine (CP) angle surgery:
  • The cochlear duct (perilymphatic duct) runs from the medial aspect of scala tympani to the subarachnoid space and terminates anteromedial to the jugular bulb and inferior to the internal auditory canal. Decompression of CSF into mastoid is an important procedure and is done by drilling medial to jugular bulb and opening of the cochlear duct in translabyrinthine approach for CP angle tumor.
- Cranial nerves 9, 10, and 11 and the inferior petrosal sinus found immediately inferior to the opening of cochlear

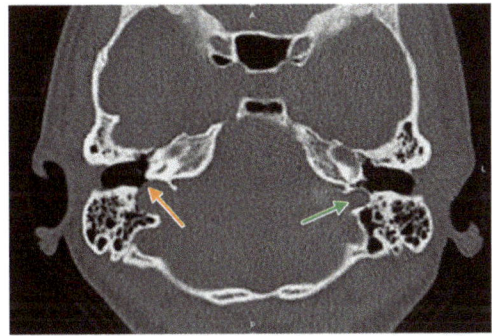

Fig. 7: Computed tomography (CT) axial cut showing dehiscent jugular bulb in the right ear. [Dehiscent jugular bulb (orange arrow); normal jugular bulb (green arrow)].

aqueduct can be used as lower limit of translabyrinthine surgery.

Lateral Wall of the Tympanic Cavity

It is formed by the tympanic bone, the tympanic membrane, and outer attic wall (scutum). It separates the external ear and the middle ear.

Lateral wall is membranous as well as bony structure. Tympanic bone at the medial end harbors the sulcus in which tympanic membrane with annulus lodges.

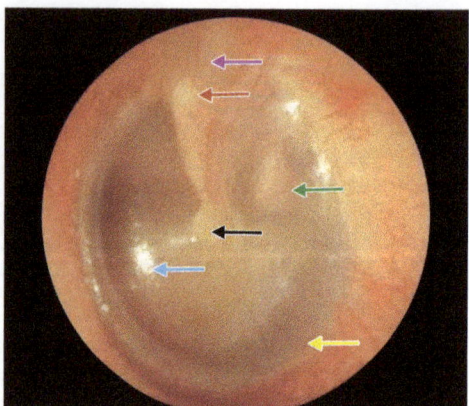

Fig. 8: Parts of a normal tympanic membrane. [Pars flaccida (purple arrow); annulus (yellow arrow); cone of light (blue arrow); lateral process of malleus (red arrow); IS joint (green arrow); umbo (black arrow)].

The conically shaped tympanic membrane **(Fig. 8)** is tilted anteroinferiorly, therefore anteroinferior bony wall is longer than posteroinferior one and anterior tympanomeatal angle is more acute than the posterior one. Adult's tympanic membrane is about 9 mm in diameter. The fibrous annulus (peripheral fibrocartilaginous part of the tympanic membrane) anchors in the tympanic sulcus (tympanic ring is C shaped and deficient part is notch of Rivinus), so annulus extends the fibrous stria from the anterior and posterior tympanic spine to the neck of malleus and forming anterior and posterior tympanic malleolar ligament which divides tympanic membrane into superior pars flaccida (Shrapnell's membrane) and inferior (pars tensa) (tympanic spine is anterosuperior and posterior superior prominent edge of the tympanic sulcus). Pars flaccida attaches to the outer wall of attic (scutum). The tympanic membrane is composed of three layers: (1) Epithelial layer, (2) fibrous layer (lamina propria), and (3) mucosal layer.

Tympanic membrane is conical in shape with its apex at umbo (at the tip of manubrium).

The tympanic membrane attaches to the malleus at the lateral process and the umbo. In between these two points there is a weak mucosal fold, the plica mallearis, which connects the tympanic membrane to the malleus.

Microscopically tympanic membrane has three layers, but it arranges differently, reflects different tensile strength of pars tensa and pars flaccida. The three canaliculi lie at the medial surface of the tympanic ring, medial to the tympanic spine and the tympanic annulus.

1. *The iter chordae anterior:* Through this opening chorda tympani exits the tympanic cavity. This opening is located at the medial end of the petrotympanic fissure.
2. *The iter chordae posterior:* Through this opening chorda tympani enters the tympanic cavity, medial to the tympanic annulus, traverses cavity with lateral to long process of incus and medial to the handle of malleus to reach up to the petrotympanic fissure.
3. *The petrotympanic fissure:* Anterior malleolar ligament, anterior tympanic artery, and the chorda tympani pass through this fissure.

Scutum or outer attic wall forms the superior part of the lateral wall. It is part of the squamous bone. The part of the attic which lies below the roof of the EAC is known as the scutum. It is a sharp bony spur where the pars flaccida is attached.

- Retraction of the pars flaccida and posterosuperior part of the pars tensa occur due to their attachment strength in organized fibers in the lamina propria.
- *Prussak's space:* The superior recess of the tympanic membrane. It is the space between the pars flaccida and the neck of malleus.
  • *Roof:* Lateral malleal fold
  • *Floor:* The neck of malleus

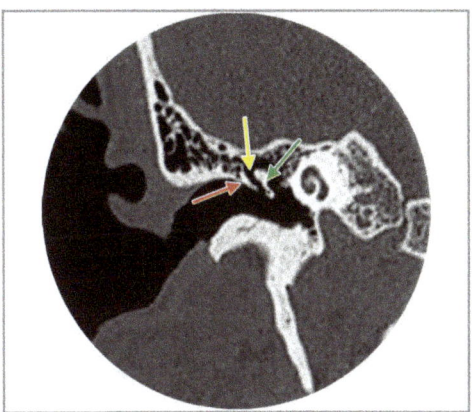

Fig. 9: Computed tomography (CT) image of the outer attic wall and Prussak's space. [Outer attic wall (red arrow); Ossicles (green arrow); Prussak's space (yellow arrow)].

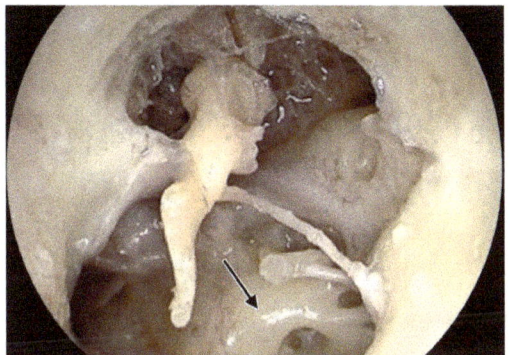

Fig. 10: Endoscopic view, promontory (arrow) on the medial wall of the middle ear.

- *Anterior wall:* Anterior malleal fold
- *Lateral wall:* Pars flaccida and the lower edge of the outer attic wall
- *Posterior wall:* Open to the posterior pouch of Von Troeltsch.

The Prussak's space **(Fig. 9)**, where epitympanic cholesteatoma starts to invaginate medially from the pars flaccida.
- Lateral wall of the tympanic membrane is the site through which clinical examination is possible for the diseases of the ear.
- As cartilaginous "cap" of the lateral process of malleus is adherent to the lamina propria of the tympanic membrane. It requires sharp, meticulous dissection to dissect the tympanic membrane in the tympanoplasty.

The Medial Wall of the Tympanic Cavity (Cochlear Wall or Surgical Floor of the Middle Ear)

The medial wall is derived from the otic capsule. It features prominent promontory with oval window and round window, cochleariformis process, tympanic segment of the facial nerve, and anterior aspect of lateral semicircular canal **(Fig. 10)**.

The promontory: It is located anteriorly to the oval window, inferiorly to the cochleariformis process. Cochlea turns around the spongy bone modiolus around 2¾ turns. Basal turn gives prominence of the promontory, middle and apical turn lies medial to the cochleariformis process and tensor tympani muscle (axis of cochlea is directed anteriorly and laterally).

The oval window and round window: The oval window is situated posterosuperior to the promontory, posterior to cochleariformis process, and the pyramidal eminence lies posteriorly, inferior to the facial nerve and covered with annular ligament and the footplate of the stapes **(Fig. 11)**.

The round window is located in the round window niche, inferiorly to the oval window and posteroinferior to the promontory. Oval window and round window are openings of the labyrinth to the tympanic cavity. True round window membrane is in horizontal plane and to see it, removal of superior overhang of niche is required.
- The superior border of the round window is very near to the basilar membrane and osseous spiral lamina.
- Intracochlear inferior border of the round window is called the "crista fenestra."

Middle Ear Cavity

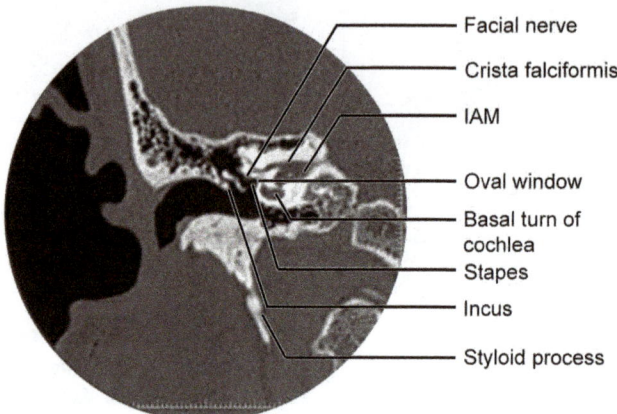

Fig. 11: Computed tomography (CT) scan axial cut showing area of stapes and oval window.

It is not closely related to the basilar membrane.

The cochleariformis process: It corresponds to the posterior end of the semicanal of tensor tympani. It is conical eminence anterosuperior to the oval window, inferior and lateral to the horizontal facial nerve. It is located just medial to the neck of malleus. The tendon of tensor tympani curves round and with right angle attaches to the neck of malleus. It is a constant landmark for the identification of the facial nerve.

The facial nerve: The tympanic segment of facial nerve courses obliquely in the medial wall of tympanic cavity from area above the supratubal recess to the area just superior to the oval window. Above the oval window, facial nerve forms prominence along with prominence of promontory, oval window lies under the level of these prominences. At the posterior edge of the oval window, facial nerve turns inferiorly and laterally from medial wall of tympanic cavity to the posterior wall of the tympanic cavity. At this turning point, facial nerve is anteroinferior to lateral semicircular canal and medial to the short process of the incus **(Fig. 12)**.

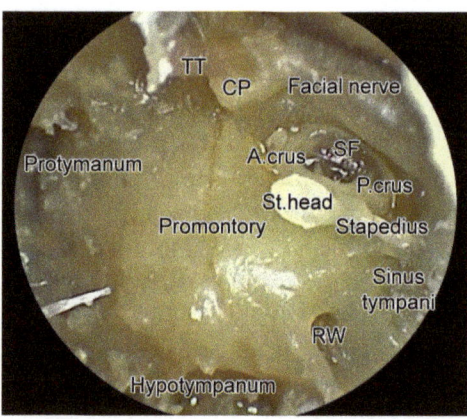

Fig. 12: Endoscopic view of the middle ear with relations of facial nerve.

Lateral Semicircular Canal (Fig. 13)

Anterior aspect of the lateral semicircular canal lies in the posterior part of the attic. The ampullae of the superior and the lateral semicircular canal are situated in the medial wall of the posterior attic.
- Anomaly of the facial nerve is associated with the anomalies of the labyrinth.
- Congenital anomalies of the oval window and the round window appear along with malformation of the labyrinth. Atresia or fixation of oval window may appear.

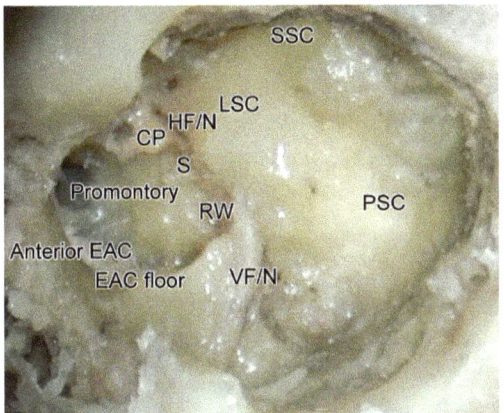

Fig. 13: Cadaveric dissection photo of mastoid with all the three superior semicircular canal (SCC).

- Cochleariformis process is constant landmark for the identification of the facial nerve.
- Facial recess approach (posterior tympanotomy) allows exposure of lower half of the basal turn of cochlea for the cochlear implant surgery.
- For exposure of middle turn and apical turn of the cochlea, cochleariformis process and the semicanal of tensor tympani must be removed.
- Oval window shows different degree of otosclerosis ranging from focal thickening to complete obliteration.
- Ampulla of posterior semicircular canal is close to the round window niche. Singular nerve supplies this ampulla. This singular canal lies immediately inferior to the posterior attachment of the round window membrane.
- *Perifenestral otosclerosis:* Round window gets obliterated in the otosclerosis and the meningitis.
- Round window membrane allows passage of the bacterial exotoxins as well as drugs such as dexamethasone and steroids into the inner ear.

The Anterior Wall of Tympanic Cavity

The anterior wall of tympanic cavity develops from otic capsule. This wall covers ICA and it contains the semicanal of Eustachian tube and semicanal of the tensor tympani muscle. A bony septum lies between the auditory tube and tensor tympani, it extends into the cochleariformis process and tensor tympani tendon rests on it. Anterior wall corresponds to the vertical segment of the ICA, medial to the semicanal of the Eustachian tube. There are two canaliculi in the bony carotid canal which transmit the superior caroticotympanic nerve and inferior caroticotympanic nerve both of which arises from superior cervical ganglion to the tympanic plexus of the middle ear.

Rarely, there is a dehiscent wall between the cochlea and carotid artery. Preoperative imaging helps to prevent inadvertent penetration into carotid during cochlear implant surgery.

The Posterior Wall of the Tympanic Cavity (Fig. 14)

This wall develops from the cartilage of the 2nd pharyngeal arch (Reichert's cartilage). The cartilaginous bar extends between the facial nerve medially to the tympanic annulus laterally. It is the highest wall of the middle ear cavity. In upper one-third, aditus ad antrum lies which connects the epitympanum to antrum. The remaining lower two-thirds of wall connects the annulus to the structure of the otic capsule containing the mastoid segment of the facial nerve. There are three eminences in the posterior wall:

1. *Pyramidal eminence:* It is triangular shape, base lies anteromedial wall of the facial nerve (mastoid). Apex gives attachment to the stapedius muscle and it transmits the nerve to stapedius, branch of facial nerve.

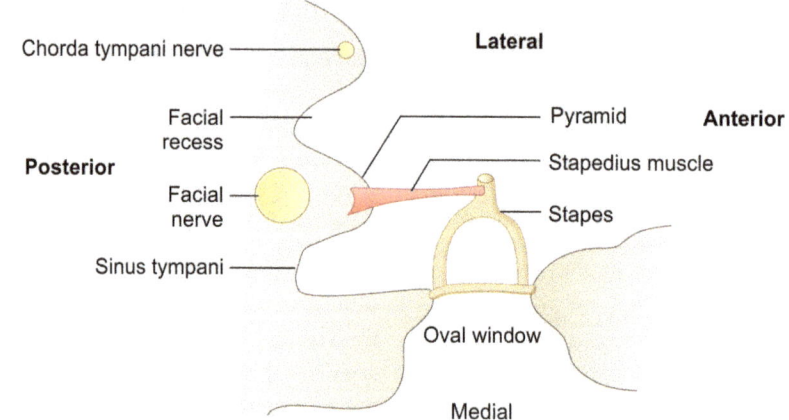

Fig. 14: Schematic diagram of posterior mesotympanum. Contents of the middle ear cavity.

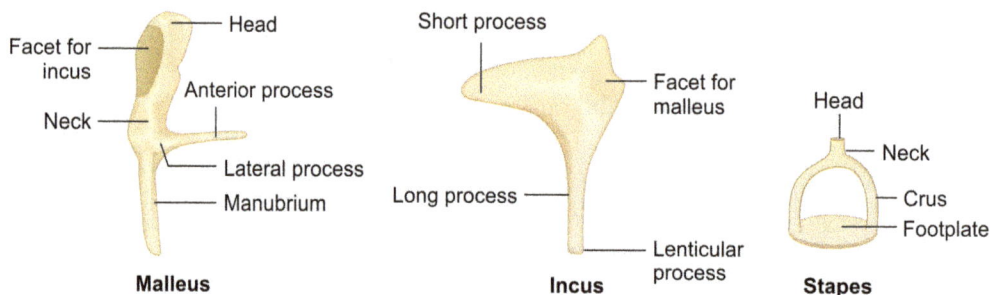

Fig. 15: Middle ear ossicles.

2. *Chordal eminence:* It lies medial to annulus and lateral to the pyramidal eminences.
3. *Styloid eminences:* It is in the inferior part of the posterior wall, represents the base of styloid process and the landmark for the facial nerve (facial nerve lies posterior to the eminence).

The middle ear cavity contains the ossicular chain with ligament and muscles. It is mucosal lining air containing cavity essential for the transmission of the sound from the tympanic membrane to the oval window.

The Ossicular Chain (Fig. 15)

The malleus, incus, and stapes resemble to their shape derived from the 1st and 2nd pharyngeal arches, respectively.

The malleus (**Fig. 16**) is the most lateral of the ossicles. It has head, neck, handle (manubrium) and processes, anterior and lateral process. The handle of malleus firmly attaches to the tympanic membrane at the lateral process and the umbo. The lateral process lies at the superolateral end of the manubrium, close to anterior canal wall, meticulous care should be taken not to touch this process with burr while performing canaloplasty. Anterior malleolar ligament and posterior incudal ligament creates the axis of ossicular rotation. The tendon of tensor tympani muscle attaches the medial side of the neck of malleus and contraction of this muscles moves the ossicles medially, tenses the tympanic membrane. There are three suspensory ligaments (anterior, lateral,

Middle Ear Cavity

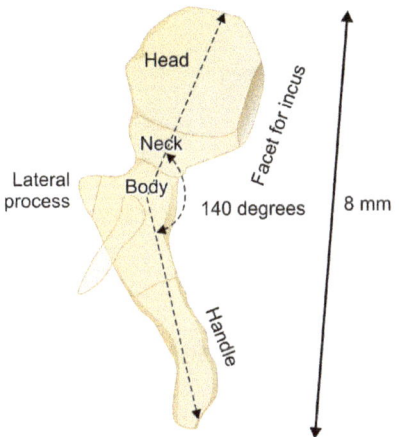

Fig. 16: Malleus.

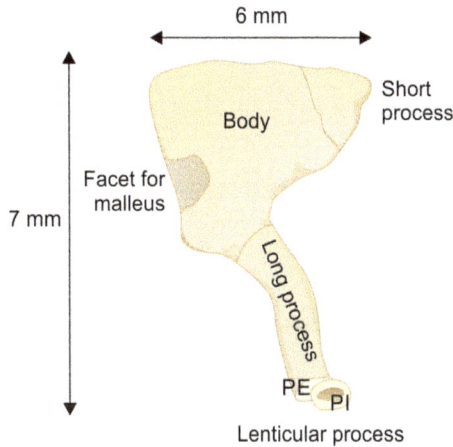

Fig. 17: Incus.

and superior) and two ligaments (anterior and posterior malleolar ligaments).

The Incus (Fig. 17)

It is largest of the three ossicles, medial to the malleus and lateral to the stapes. It has body (articulate with head of malleus), long process, short process, and lenticular process (articulate with the head of stapes).

The head of malleus and body of incus lie in the epitympanum. Short process of incus lies over the incudal butress. Long process lies parallel and slight medial to manubrium articulate as lenticular process to the head of stapes. The incus has three ligaments.

The Stapes (Fig. 18)

The smallest and the most medial of the ossicles. The head, neck, two unequal crura, and the footplate. The stapedius muscle develops from the 2nd pharyngeal arch and supplied by the facial nerve, attaches to the neck of the stapes and the footplate reaccommodates into the oval window by stapediovestibular ligament (annular ligament). A contraction of the stapedius muscles tilts the stapes and its footplate resulting in tension in the annular ligament limits sound transmission to the inner ear.

- The osteolytic changes affect the incus first (lenticular and long process).
- The malleus and the footplate are more resistant to necrosis.
- Aseptic necrosis of the stapes occurs due to retracted tympanic membrane or over crimpled prosthesis of the stapes.
- In stapes surgery, to prevent subluxation of the footplate. It is safe to cut the posterior crus than fracture.
- In otosclerosis, in early-stage osteosclerotic foci involves anterior aspect the annular ligament. It impairs the piston-like movement (unaffecting the rocking movement), hence, causing the low frequency sensorineural deafness.
- The conductive hearing impairment as a result of malleus fixation depends upon location, extent, and type of pathology causing fixation.
- Calcification of anterior malleal ligament results in hearing loss <10 dB, more commonly fixation of head by bony spur (to tegmen tympani/lateral attic wall) causes 15–20 dB hearing loss.

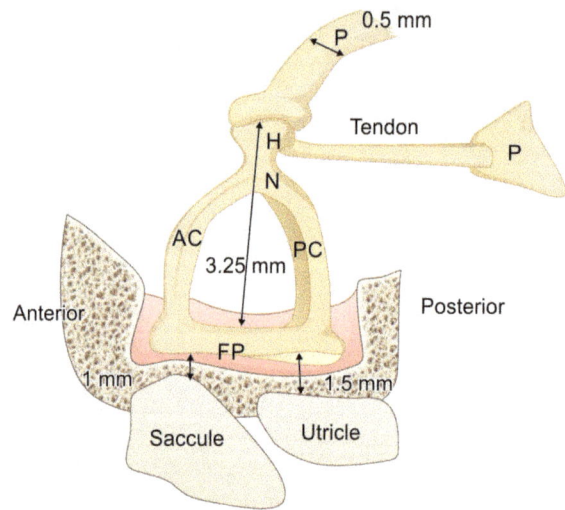

Fig. 18: Stapes. (Stapes in the oval window niche and its relationship with the underlying saccule and utricle; *: annular ligament; P: pyramidal eminence; H: head; N: neck; AC: anterior crus; PC: posterior crus; FP: foot plate)

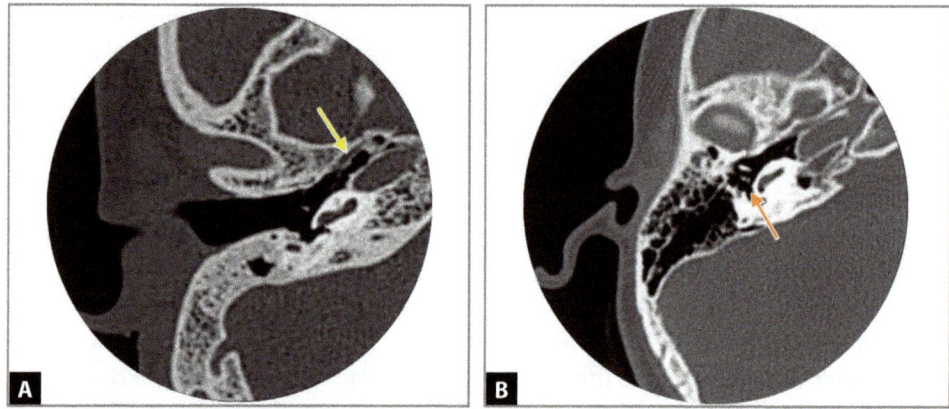

Figs. 19A and B: (A) Computed tomography (CT) axial cut showing tensor tympani muscle; (B) Computed tomography (CT) scan axial cut showing stapedius muscle. [Tensor tymapni muscle (yellow arrow); stapedius muscle (orange arrow)].

- Incudomalleal and incudostapedial joints are lined with cartilage. These joints have true capsule lined with synovial membrane.

Middle Ear Muscles (Figs. 19A and B)

The tensor tympani muscle develops from the first brachial arch, supplied by trigeminal nerve and arises from the walls of its semicanal, greater wing of sphenoid and cartilage of the auditory tube. The tendon of the tensor tympani muscle curves around the cochleariformis process and inserted into neck of malleus.

The stapedius runs in vertical plane and attaches the apex of the pyramidal eminence (anteromedial to mastoid segment of facial nerve). The posterior crus receives innervations from the facial nerve.

Nerves of the Tympanic Cavity

Jacobson's Nerve

It is tympanic branch of inferior ganglion of the 9th glossopharyngeal nerve located at jugulocarotid crest, enters the tympanic cavity near the medial wall of hypotympanum through hypotympanic fissure with branch of inferior tympanic artery and it ascends the medial wall and reaches the promontory. It unites with caroticotympanic branch at the promontory and forms the tympanic plexus. Union of preganglionic fibers of Jacobson's nerve and postganglionic fibers of the caroticotympanic nerve give rise to lesser petrosal nerve which ascends upward beneath the semicanal of the tensor tympani muscle and exit the tympanic cavity at subcanal sulcus to reach the floor of middle cranial fossa (facial hiatus).

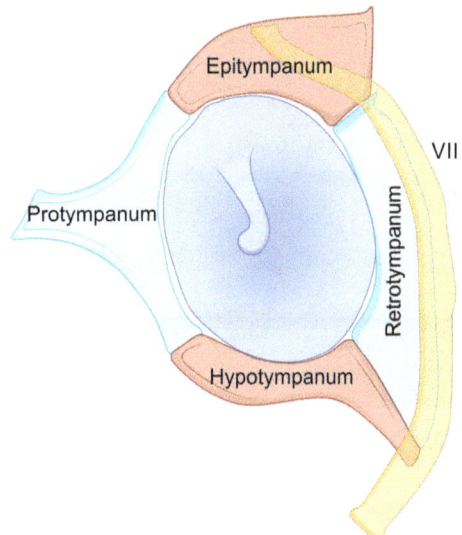

Fig. 20: Compartments of the middle ear. (VII: facial nerve)

Arnold's Nerve

This nerve has fibers of auricular branch 10th nerve with facial, glossopharyngeal, and vagus nerve. Through mastoid canaliculus, it enters the fallopian canal. Involvement of the EAC shows involvement of Arnold's nerve in herpetic infections. Cough reflex is elicited by manipulation of EAC.

Middle Ear Blood Vessels

Branches from the external carotid arteries contribute to the arterial network of the middle ear. Anterior tympanic artery, deep auricular artery, mastoid artery, stylomastoid artery, superficial petrosal artery, and tubal artery supply the area.

The tympanic cavity is divided into the epitympanum, mesotympanum, protympanum, hypotympanum, and retrotympanum (**Fig. 20**).

Epitympanum

It is the upper part of the tympanic cavity which lies above the horizontal line passing at the neck of malleus. It contains the head of malleus and body of incus.

- Superior wall—tegmen tympani
- Anterior wall—zygomatic arch
- Posterior—opens into aditus an antrum
- Medial wall—(petrous bone) horizontal part of facial nerve and lateral semicircular canal with supralabyrinthine air cells within medial wall
- Lateral wall—scutum and pars flaccida.

The epitympanum divides into anterior and posterior epitympanum by the cog. Anterior epitympanum is again divided into the anterior malleolar space and anterior epitympanic recess. This recess is connected to the protympanum by supratubal recess (**Fig. 21**). The posterior epitympanum contains the head of malleus and body of incus.

Mesotympanum

It is the largest compartment of tympanic cavity medial to pars tensa. Mesotympanum communicates with epitympanum through

Middle Ear Cavity

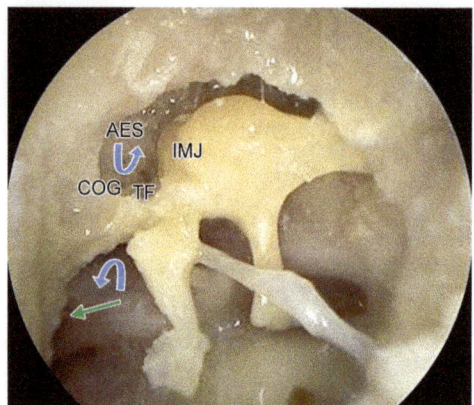

Fig. 21: Endoscopic diagram showing supratubal recess (green arrow).

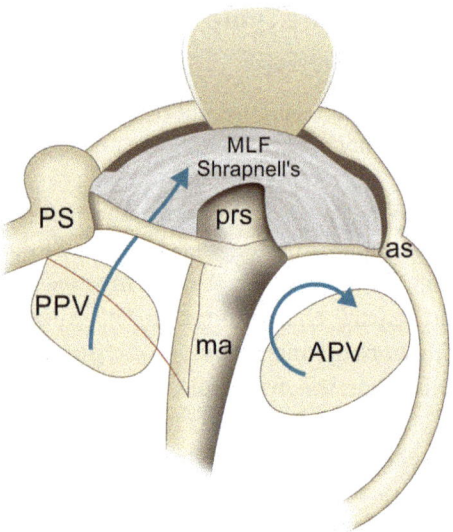

Fig. 22: Anterior and posterior pouch of Von Troeltsch. (Right middle ear lateral wall compartments after removal of the pars tensa, showing the anterior pouch of Von Troeltsch (APV) that is isolated Prussk's space and the posterior pouch of Von Troeltsch (PPV) that is in communication with the Prussak's space; as: anterior tympanic spine; ps: posterior tympanic spine; ma: malleus handle)

anterior and posterior pouch of Von Troeltsch **(Fig. 22)** (space between the malleolar fold and the tympanic membrane).

Hypotympanum

It is a part of middle ear cavity which lies below tympanic cavity.
- Lateral wall—tympanic bone
- Medial wall—formed by petrous bone and lower part formed by infracochlear hypotympanic air cells
- Anterior wall—part of petrous bone separates ICA
- Posterior wall—styloid eminence and lower part of facial nerve
- Inferior wall—separates it from jugular bulb.

Retrofacial Air Cells

Cells from the central mastoid extend medial to the facial nerve and drain into hypotympanic space.

Protympanum

The part of the middle ear that lies anterior to the anterior margin of tympanic membrane. It contains Eustachian tube.

- Lateral wall—thin plate of tympanic bone separates it from the mandibular fossa
- Medial wall—cochlea posteriorly
- ICA anteriorly
- Roof—semicanal of the tensor tympani and tensor tympani fold separates it from the anterior attic.

Supratubal Recess

Superior extension of the protympanum lying between the tensor tympani fold and superior border of Eustachian tube.

Retrotympanum

This compartment or space lies posterior and medial to the tympanic annulus. It has the highest rate of the middle ear disease because of hidden spaces within. The retrotympanum

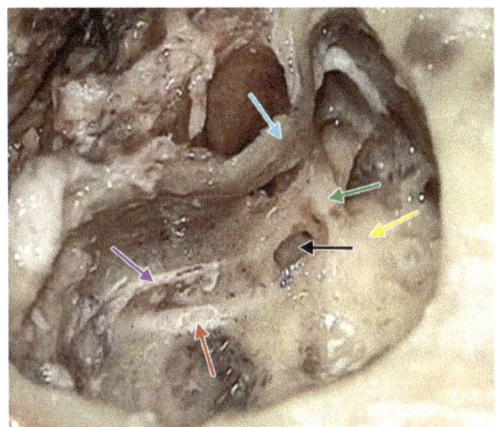

Fig. 23: Microscopic dissection image showing facial recess and its boundaries. [Posterior EAC (blue arrow); incus buttress (green arrow); LSC (yellow arrow); chordatympani (purple arrow); vertical facial nerve (red arrow); facial recess (black arrow)].

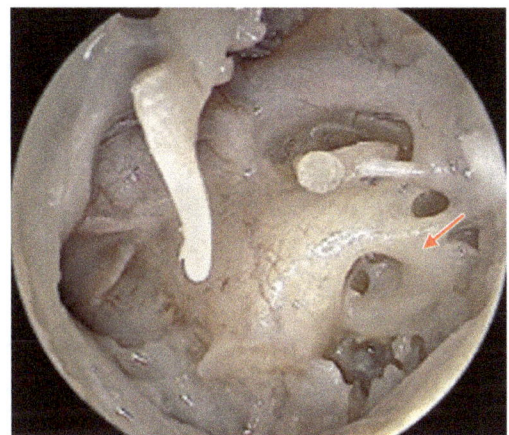

Fig. 24: Endoscopic view of middle ear showing sinus tympani.

includes four spaces—two medial to the facial nerve and two lateral to the facial nerve. Facial recess, sinus tympani, posterior tympanic sinus, and lateral tympanic sinus are spaces which lie within retrotympanum.

Facial Recess (Fig. 23)

Its lateral part is bounded anterolaterally by the chorda tympani, posteromedially by the vertical facial nerve and superiorly by the incudal buttress (short process of incus rests on it). Facial recess divides into two parts— (1) facial sinus (superior), and (2) lateral tympanic sinus (inferior).

The size of facial recess acquires adult configuration at the time of birth. Facial recess approaches in transmastoid approach allows to visualize the sinus tympani, oval window, round window, promontory and hypotympanic air cells. Extended facial recess approach is acquired by sacrificing the chorda tympani nerve.

Medial spaces are the posterior tympanic sinus and the sinus tympani (**Fig. 24**). It is the space lying medial to the facial nerve and pyramid eminence, lateral to the labyrinth and posterior to the promontory.

The ponticulus is bony ridge from the promontory to the pyramidal eminence and subiculum is the bony ridge from the styloid eminence to the posterior pillar of the round window niche.

Spaces above the ponticulus are known as posterior tympanic sinus which lies beneath (medial to the stapedius muscle and pyramidal eminence).

To clear disease from the posterior tympanic sinus, drilling of the pyramidal eminence and stapedius muscle has to be cut.

Sinus Tympani

It is a hidden space, medial to the mastoid segment of the facial nerve. It is a frequent site for the recurrence of cholesteatoma. It lies between ponticulus (promontory to the pyramidal process) and subiculum (bony ridge from the styloid eminence to the posterior pillar of the round window niche). This space lies between vertical segment of facial nerve, pyramidal eminence, stapedius muscle (tendon) laterally, and the vestibule and posterior semicircular canal medially.

Types of the Sinus Tympani

- *Small sinus tympani:* The posterior and medial boundaries of the space extend only up to anterior edge of the vertical facial nerve.
- *Deep sinus tympani:* The posterior and medial limit passes the posterior edge of vertical facial nerve.
- *Deep sinus with posterior extension:* The posterior and medial limit passes the posterior edge of vertical facial nerve, Retrofacial (medial to facial nerve) requires reaching this large space. Cholesteatoma may be removed using angled instruments with an endoscopic technique in this type of sinus tympani.

Recognition of the spaces of retrotympanum is mandatory to remove the cholesteatoma debris without injury to the structures of posterior mesotympanum (stapes, round window, dehiscent, or high jugular bulb).

BIBLIOGRAPHY

1. Adad B, Ragson BM, Ackerson L. Relationship of the facial nerve to the tympanic annulus: a direct anatomic examination. Laryngoscope. 1999;109:1189-92.
2. Alberti PW. The blood supply of the long process of the incus and the head and neck of stapes. J Laryngol Otol. 1965;79:966-70.
3. Anson BJ, Caulowell EW. The developmental anatomy of the human stapes. Ann Otol Rhinol Laryngol. 1942;51:891-904.
4. Carfrae MJ, Jahrsdoerfer RA, Kesser BW. Malleus bar: an unusual ossicular abnormality in the setting of congenital aural atresia. Otol Neurotol. 2010;31(3):415-8.
5. Chien W, Northrop C, Levine S, Pilch BZ, Peake WT, Rosowski JJ, et al. Anatomy of the distal incus in humans. J Assoc Res Otolaryngol. 2009;10(4):485-96.
6. Davies DG. Malleus fixation. J Laryngol Otol. 1968;82:331-51.
7. Eby TL. Development of the facial recess: implications for cochlear implantation. Laryngoscope. 1996;106(5 Pt 2 Suppl 80):1-7.
8. Friedmann DR, Eubig J, McGill M, Babb JS, Pramanik BK, Lalwani AK. Development of the jugular bulb: a radiologic study. Otol Neurotol. 2011;32(8):1389-95.
9. Friedmann DR, Le BT, Pramanik BK, Lalwani AK. Clinical spectrum of patients with erosion of the inner ear by jugular bulb abnormalities. Laryngoscope. 2010;120(2):365-72.
10. Funasaka S. Congenital ossicular anomalies without malformations of the external ear. Arch Otorhinolaryngol. 1979;224:231-40.
11. Funnell W, Robert J, Heng Siah T, McKee Marc D, Daniel SJ, Decraemer WF. On the coupling between the incus and the stapes in the cat. J Assoc Res Otolaryngol. 2005;6:9-18.
12. Graham MD. The jugular bulb: its anatomic and clinical considerations in contemporary otology. Laryngoscope. 1977;87(1):105-25.
13. Henson Jr OW, Henson MM. The tympanic membrane: highly developed smooth muscle arrays in the annulus fibrosus of mustached bats. J Assoc Res Otolaryngol. 2000;1:25-32.
14. Herman HK, Kimmelman CP. Congenital anomalies limited to the middle ear. Otolaryngol Head Neck Surg. 1992;106:285-7.
15. Jaskoll F. Morphogensis and teratogenesis of the middle ear in animals. Birth Defects Orig Artic Ser. 1980;XVI(7):9-28.
16. Kurosaki Y, Tanaka YO, Itai Y. Malleus bar as a rare cause of congenital malleus fixation: CT demonstration. AJNR Am J Neuroradiol. 1998;19:1229-30.
17. Langman J. Embryologie Médicale. Paris: Masson; 1965. p. 34.
18. Lannigan FJ, O'Higgins P, McPhie P. The vascular supply of the lenticular and long processes of the incus. Clin Otolaryngol Allied Sci. 1993;18:387-9.
19. Lim DJ. Structure and function of the tympanic membrane: a review. Acta Otorhinolaryngol Belg. 1995;49:101-15.
20. Lim DJ. Tympanic membrane: electron microscopic observations, part I: pars tensa. Acta Otolaryngol. 1968;66:181-98.

21. Lim DJ. Tympanic membrane: electron microscopic observations, part II: pars fláccida. Acta Otolaryngol. 1968;66(3):515-32.
22. Louryan S. Pure second branchial arch syndrome. Ann Otol Rhinol Laryngol. 1993;102:904-5.
23. Makino K, Amatsu M. Epithelial migration on the tympanic membrane and external canal. Arch Otorhinolaryngol. 1986;243(1):39-42.
24. Mansour S, Nicolas K, Sbeity S. Triple ossicular fixation and semicircular canal malformations. J Otolaryngol. 2007;36(3): E31-4.
25. Martin JF, Bradley A, Olson EN. The paired-like homeo box gene MHox is required for early events of skeletogenesis in multiple lineages. Genes Dev. 1995;9:1237-49.
26. Michaels L. An epidermoid formation in the developing middle ear: a possible source of cholesteatoma. J Otolaryngol. 1986;15(3): 169-74.
27. Michaels L. Origin of congenital cholesteatoma from a normally occurring epidermoid rest in the developing middle ear. Int J Pediatr Otorhinolaryngol. 1988;15(1):51-65.
28. Miklós Tóth, Pre- and postnatal changes in the human tympanic cavity, Semmelweis University School of Doctoral Studies for Developmental Biology Ph.D. Thesis, Budapest; 2007.
29. Nandapalan V, Tos M. Isolated congenital stapes ankylosis: an embryologic survey and literature review. Am J Otol. 2000;21(1):71-80.
30. Palva T, Johnsson LG. Epitympanic compartment surgical considerations: reevaluation. Am J Otol. 1995;16(4):505-13.
31. Paço J, Branco C, Estibeiro H, Oliveira E, Carmo D. The posterosuperior quadrant of the tympanic membrane. Otolaryngol Head Neck Surg. 2009;140(6):884-8.
32. Rodriguez K, Shah RK, Kenna M. Anomalies of the middle and inner ear. Otolaryngol Clin North Am. 2007;40(1):81-96, vi.
33. Roland Jr JT, Hoffman RA, Miller PJ, Cohen NL. Retrofacial approach to the hypotympanum. Arch Otolaryngol Head Neck Surg. 1995;121(2):233-6.
34. Sadé J. Retraction pockets and attic cholesteatomas. Acta Otorhinolaryngol Belg. 1980;34(1):62-84.
35. Sanna M, Fois P, Paolo F, Russo A, Falcioni M. Management of meningoencephalic herniation of the temporal bone: personal experience and literature review. Laryngoscope. 2009;119:1579-85.
36. Shrapnell HJ. On the form and structure of the membrane timpani. London Med Gazette. 1832;10:120-4.
37. Spector GJ, Ge XX. Development of the hypotympanum in the human fetus and neonate. Ann Otol Rhinol Laryngol Suppl. 1981;90(6 Pt 2):1-20.
38. Swartz JD, Wolfson RJ, Marlowe FI, Popky GL. Postinflammatory ossicular fixation: CT analysis with surgical correlation. Radiology. 1985;154:697-700.
39. Tabb HG. Symposium: congenital anomalies of the middle ear. I. Epitympanic fixation of incus and malleus. Laryngoscope. 1976;86(2): 243-6.
40. Watson C. Necrosis of the incus by the chorda tympani nerve. J Laryngol Otol. 1992;106:252-3.
41. Wengen DF, Nishihara S, Kurokawa H, Goode RL. Measurements of stapes super structure. Ann Otol Rhinol Laryngol. 1995;104:311-6.

CHAPTER 3

Middle Ear Compartment

SURGICAL ANATOMY OF THE TYMPANOMASTOID COMPARTMENTS

Embryogenic Route of Cholesteatoma Growth

The majority of cholesteatoma follows fairly typical patterns of growth dictated by their site of origin and its related anatomic structures. The most common sites for the cholesteatoma are the posterior epitympanum, the mesotympanum, and the anterior epitympanum. Spread of cholesteatoma is along the vestigial planes that were created during the development of the ear.

During development, in tubotympanic recess, four endothelial lined sacs evaginate from the first branchial pouch to form the tympanic cavity (**Flowchart 1**). Mucosal folds and ossicular suspensory ligaments are formed where these sacs contact each other. These define various pouches, spaces, and compartments (tympanic diaphragm and tympanic isthmus) that divide the middle ear.

There are four sacci (**Fig. 1**)
1. Saccus anticus
2. Saccus medius
3. Saccus superior
4. Saccus posticus.

Saccus Anticus

The saccus anticus is the smallest saccule. It forms the anterior pouch of Von Troeltsch and anterior epitympanic recess. At the tensor tympani muscle canal, anterior saccule of saccus medius and saccus anticus fuses and forms the tensor tympani fold, which separates the anterior epitympanic recess superiorly from the supratubal recess inferiorly.

Saccus Medius

The saccus medius forms the attic. It extends upwards and divides into three saccules:
1. *Anterior saccule:* It develops upward to form the anterior compartment of the attic.
2. *Medial saccule:* It forms superior incudal space by its growth over the incudomalleal bodies and the posterior incudal ligament.

   The Prussak's space is created by forward offshoot of the medial saccule of saccus medius.
3. *Posterior saccule:* It forms the medial portion of the mastoid antrum derived from the petrous part of the temporal bone by extending posteriorly between the long process of incus and the stapes.

Saccus Superior

It forms the inferior incudal space and posterior pouch of the Von Troeltsch. It extends posteriorly and laterally, between the handle of malleus and the long process of incus, forms the lateral part of the antrum which is derived from the squamous part of

Middle Ear Compartment

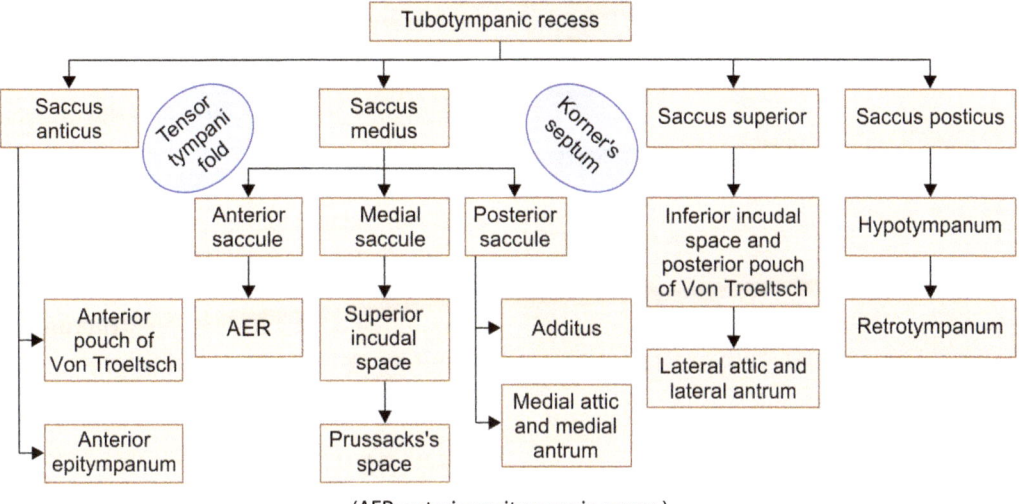

Flowchart 1: The embryology of the middle ear spaces.

(AER: anterior epitympanic recess)

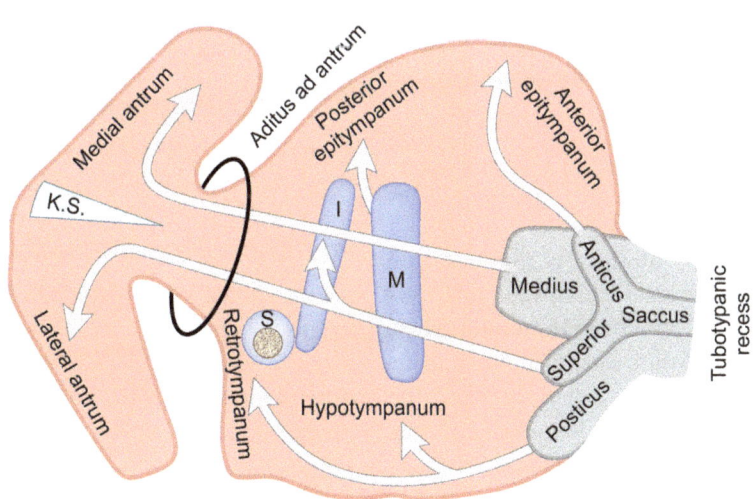

Fig. 1: The embryology of the middle ear spaces. (I; incus; M: malleus; S: stapes; K.S.: Korner's septum)

the temporal bone. A bony septum persists between the saccus superior and posterior part of the saccus medius. Breakdown fails, then bony septum in this area is known as Korner's septum **(Fig. 2)**.

Saccus Posticus

It extends along the hypotympanum and posteriorly forms the round window, the oval window, the facial recess, and the sinus tympani.

TYPICAL SPREAD OF CHOLESTEATOMA

Posterior Epitympanic Cholesteatoma

The most common route of cholesteatoma penetrates from the Prussak's space to the

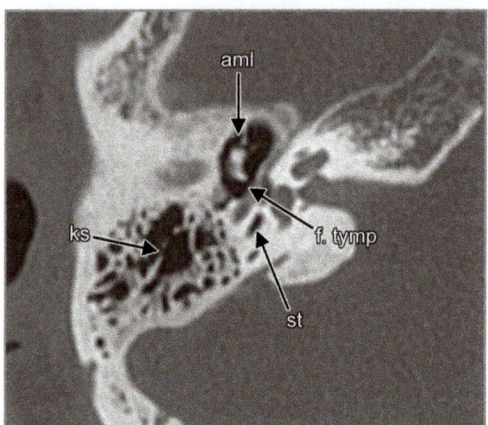

Fig. 2: Computed tomography (CT) scan axial showing the Korner's septum.

superior incudal space (lateral to incudal body) traverses the aditus ad antrum to enter the mastoid. The posterior epitympanic cholesteatoma enters the middle ear through the posterior pouch of the Von Troeltsch.

Posterior Mesotympanic Cholesteatoma

Posterior mesotympanic cholesteatoma extends to the mastoid through posterior tympanic isthmus and inferior incudal space. It passes to the mastoid, medial to the malleus and the incus. The sinus tympani and the facial recess are commonly involved (contrast to the posterior epitympanum).

Anterior Epitympanic Cholesteatoma

Epitympanic retraction occurs anterior to the malleus head, which may easily be overlooked during the tympanomastoidectomy. Anteroinferior extension to the supratubal recess is common. Cholesteatoma extends to the mesotympanum by the anterior pouch of Von Troeltsch.

A series of mucosal folds **(Figs. 3A and B)**, suspensory ligaments along with the ossicular chain known as the tympanic diaphragm: These folds are not a true barrier against the extension of disease. There are composite fold and duplicate folds. The composite folds are combination of ligament and lining mucosa with free edge. It carries blood vessels, for example, anterior malleal ligament fold and posterior incudal fold.

Duplicate folds: Thin mucosal structure arising from the fusion of expanding air sac wall without intervening structure, for example, tensor tympani fold and lateral incudomalleal fold.

FOLDS RELATED TO THE MALLEUS

Anterior Tympanomalleal Fold (Fig. 4)

It extends from the anterior tympanic spine to the anterior part of the neck of malleus. It forms the medial wall of the anterior pouch of Von Troeltsch.

Posterior Tympanomalleal Fold

It extends from the posterior tympanic spine to the posterior part of the neck of malleus. It fuses with downturn of the anterior portion of lateral incudomalleal fold. It forms the medial wall of the posterior pouch of Von Troeltsch.

Anterior Malleal Ligament

It forms the anterior limit of Prussak's space. It reflected from the anterior part of neck of the malleus to the scutum.

Lateral Malleal Ligamental Fold

Thick fold extends from the middle of the neck of malleus to the anterior attic wall. It forms the roof of Prussak's space. The defect of this fold provides direct communications between the upper and lower lateral unit.

Middle Ear Compartment

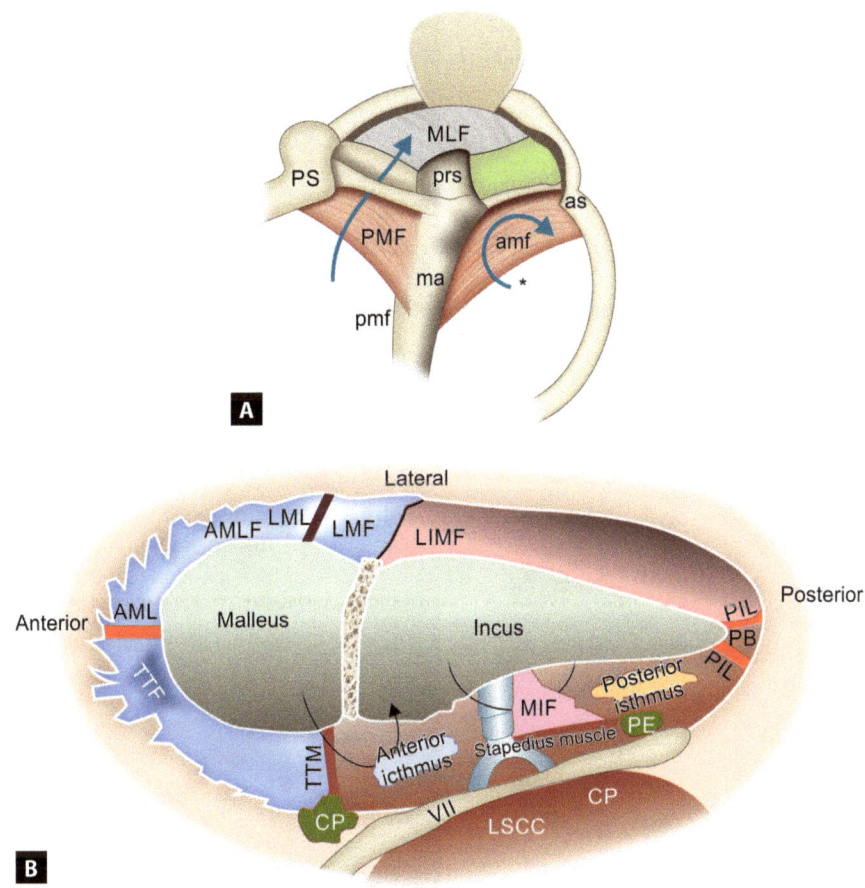

Figs. 3A and B: (A) The various middle ear folds; (B) The middle ear folds from the superior view of the epitympanum. [(Lateral view of a right middle ear after removal of the tympanic membrane; amf: anterior malleal fold; pmf: posterior malleal fold; as: anterior tympanic spine; ps: posterior tympanic spine; Arrow: root of ventilation of a Prussak's space; prs: Prussak's space; *: complete closure of the Prussak's space floor anteriorly; ma: manubrium). (Superior view of right middle ear showing the tympanic diaphragm and tympanic isthmus. Arrow: normal route of attic aeration from the mesotympanum, AMLF: anterior malleal ligament fold; TTF: tensor tympanic fold; LMF: lateral malleal fold; LIMF: lateral incudomalleal fold; AML: anterior malleal ligament; LML: lateral malleal ligament; PIL: posterior incudal ligament; TTM: tensor tympanic muscle tendon; CP: cochlearifom process; PE: pyramidal eminence; LSCC: lateral semicircular canal; PB: petrous bone)]

Superior Malleal Ligamental Fold (Fig. 5)

This fold is in the transverse plane, extends from the head of malleus to the tegmen tympani. It divides epitympanum into anterior and posterior epitympanum.

■ FOLDS RELATED TO THE INCUS
Superior Incudal Fold

It extends from the body of the incus to the tegmen tympani and divides the posterior epitympanum into the lateral posterior and medial posterior attic.

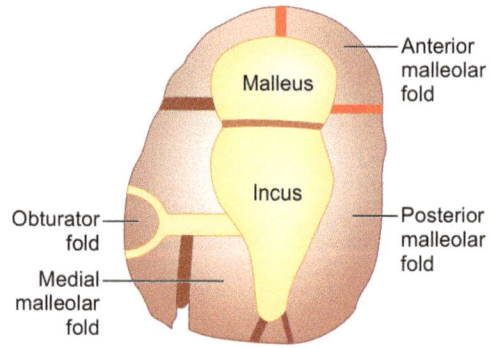

Fig. 4: Anterior malleolar fold.

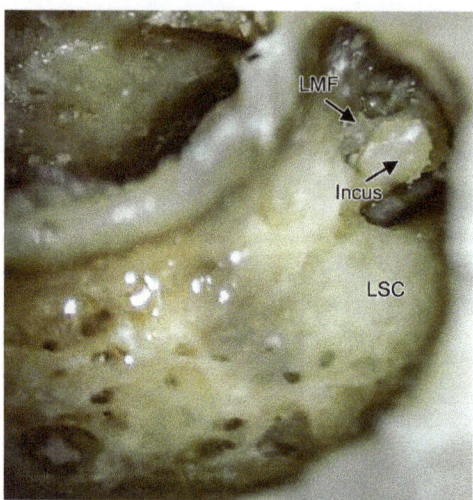

Fig. 6: Cadaveric dissection showing lateral malleolar fold.

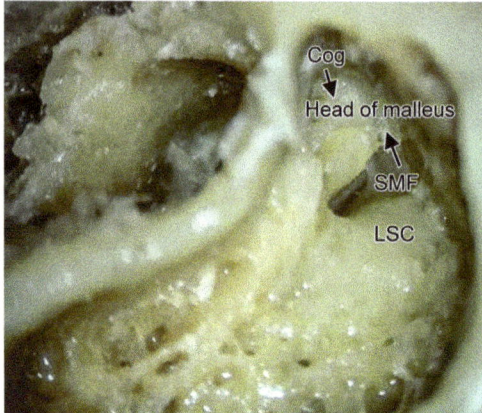

Fig. 5: Cadaveric dissection showing superior malleolar fold.

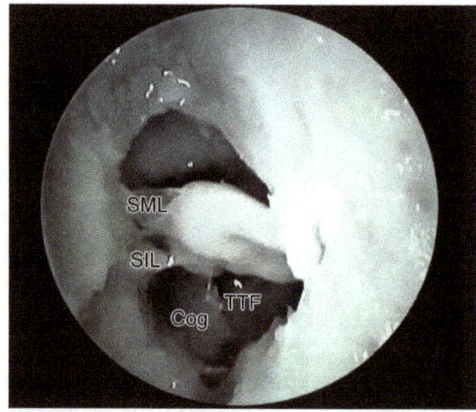

Fig. 7: Endoscopic view of ear showing tensor tympani fold. (SML: superior malleolar fold; SIL: superior incudal fold; TTF: tensor tympani fold).

Posterior Incudal Fold

It runs between fibers of the posterior incudal ligament.

Lateral Incudomalleal Fold (Fig. 6)

In relation to the lateral malleal ligament, it divides the lateral attic compartment (posterior) into the upper and lower lateral attic. It attaches posteriorly to the body of the incus and incudomalleal joint medially and laterally it attaches to the medial surface of the scutum. The anterior portion of the fold merges with the posterior portion of the lateral malleal ligament representing the posterior limit of the lateral malleal space.

Tensor Tympani Fold (Fig. 7)

It arises posteriorly from the tensor tympani tendon and runs anteriorly toward the anterior wall of attic, inserting into transverse crest and supratubal ridge. Medially, it inserts on the bony canal. Laterally it inserts on the anterior malleal ligament. The lateral part of the fold is related to the anterior portion of the chorda tympani.

If it is complete, it leads to complete separation of the anterior epitympanum and the protympanum. If it is incomplete, protympanum is confluent with the anterior epitympanum. This incomplete fold allows direct communication from the Eustachian tube and ventilating the entire attic.

All these folds with ossicular chain form the tympanic diaphragm. The tympanic diaphragm is not truly horizontal. It separates the upper unit of the attic from the mesotympanum and the lower unit of the attic, the Prussak's space inferiorly.

The Tympanic Isthmus

The mastoid and epitympanum are separated from the mesotympanum by the diaphragm. The attic is ventilated through the tympanic isthmus. The Prussak's space is ventilated through the posterior pouch of Von Troeltsch. Tympanic isthmus extends from the tensor tympani anteriorly to the posterior incudal ligament posterosuperiorly and pyramidal eminence posteroinferiorly. The distance between the tensor tympani muscle to the anterior edge of the posterior incudal ligament is around 6 mm. The isthmus is bounded laterally by the malleus head, incus and medially by the medial wall of the attic.

The anterior isthmus is the most important. It is situated between the tensor tympani anteriorly and the stapes posteroinferiorly.

Posterior tympanic isthmus is less important, situated between the short process of the incus and the stapedius muscle.

The epitympanum divides into the small anterior and large posterior compartment by the superior malleal fold. Anterior epitympanic compartment divides into the anterior malleal space and anterior epitympanic recess by "The Cog."

The posterior epitympanic compartment divides into lateral and medial part by the superior incudal fold. Lateral incudomalleal and lateral malleal fold divide lateral posterior attic into the upper lateral (superior incudal space) and lower lateral (inferior incudal space) attic compartment.

The patency of the tympanic isthmus and aditus ad antrum is important for aeration of the mastoid. Inflammatory condition of the tympanic cavity can block this ventilatory route, negative pressure develops in the mastoid and followed by exudation, granulation, chronic infection, or cholesterol granuloma. Thus, cholesteatoma confined to middle ear may give rise to chronic infection (or spread of disease) in the mastoid even it is not directly involved by the disease. It is frequently a goal in chronic ear surgery to maximize the opening between the middle ear and the mastoid.

The Mastoid

The mastoid name is derived from the Greek word "The Masto's" in reference to its shape. The mastoid process projects from the base of skull. In the temporal bone, it is situated posterior to the external auditory canal (EAC), at inferior part of the outer surface of the temporal bone. It is a bulbous, bony structure shaped by the expansion of air-filled space (pneumatization) within. The constant pull of the sternocleidomastoid muscle and posterior belly of the digastric muscle elongates the mastoid inferiorly to form the mastoid tip or mastoid process.

The mastoid process appears at the 29th week of gestation due to fusion of the bone of the otic capsule with the squamous bone. At birth, it is underdeveloped and becomes prominent by 2 years of age and continues to grow till 6 years. Endothelial lined sac replaces the mesenchyme of the mastoid bone. This process is known as pneumatization. So, air-containing mastoid cavity is known as mastoid air cells **(Fig. 8; Flowchart 2)**.

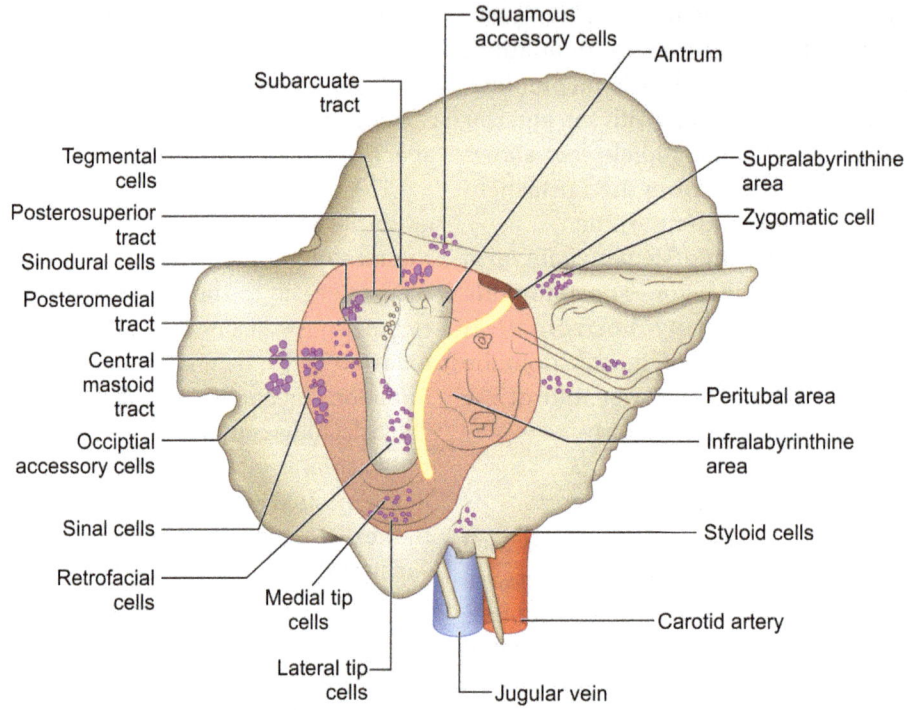

Pneumatization of the temporal bone with regions areas and tracts indicated

Fig. 8: Various mastoid air cells.

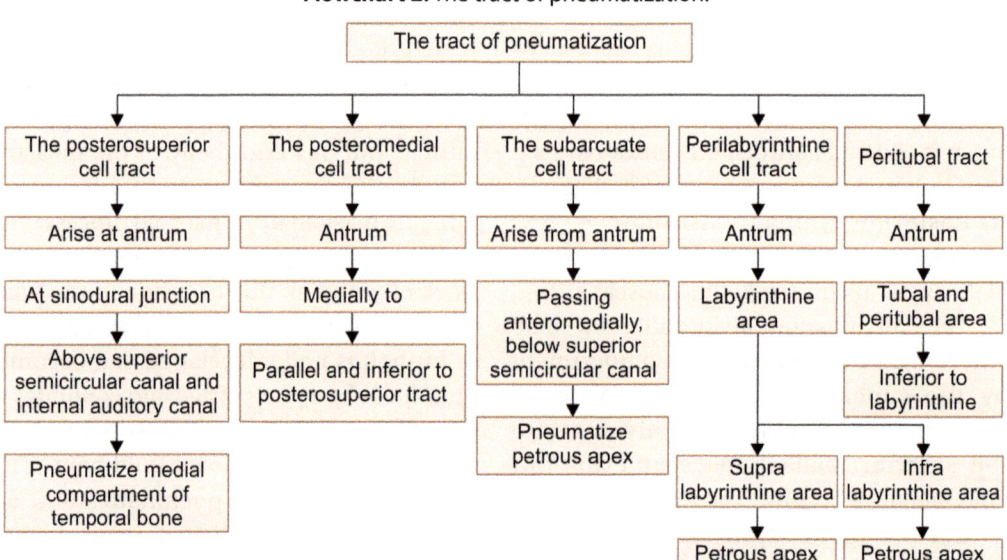

Middle Ear Compartment

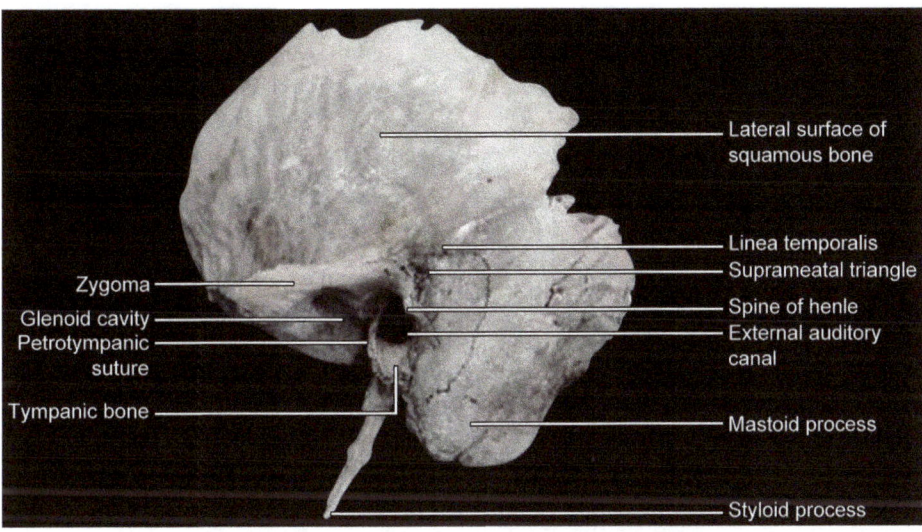

Fig. 9: Lateral surface with important landmarks.

The mastoid antrum is the biggest air cell. Mastoid antrum reaches adult size by birth. In postnatal period, epithelial air tract buds from the antrum extend to the adjacent area and forms the mastoid air cells.

- The mastoid antrum, medial to the MacEwen triangle, develops in the earliest stages of mastoid pneumatization and is always present in even at the least pneumatized temporal bones. Therefore, the fossa mastoidea is the site at which mastoid drilling ordinarily commences.
- Lateral surface of the mastoid **(Fig. 9)** has important landmark, temporal line, Henle's spine, and MacEwen triangle.
- Digastric groove on the inner surface of the mastoid tip is constant guide to the facial nerve exit from a stylomastoid foramen.

Mastoid Antrum and Deeper Structures (Fig. 10)

- The lateral semicircular canal lies in the floor of the mastoid antrum.
- Superior semicircular canal is perpendicular and medial to the lateral semicircular canal.

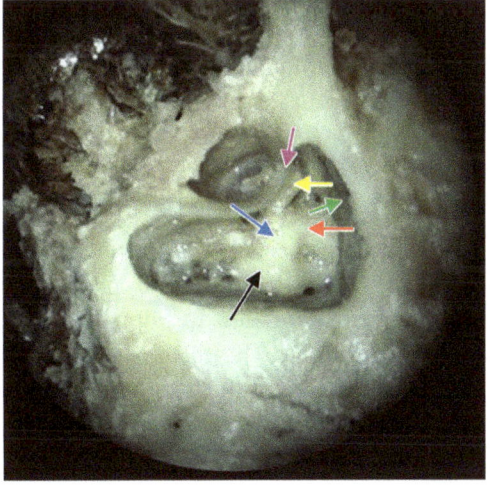

Fig. 10: Deep relations of the mastoid antrum. [Posterior EAC (purple arrow); short process of incus (yellow arrow); MCF dura (green arrow); superior SCC (red arrow); lateral SCC (blue arrow); posterior SCC (black arrow)].

- Posterior semicircular canal is also perpendicular and superior to the Donaldson's line (it is a straight line that turns in the axis of the horizontal semicircular canal and bisects the posterior semicircular canal).

- The endolymphatic sac is inferior and medial to this line. Surgical exposure is possible through retrofacial approach, area is bounded by sigmoid sinus, posterior semicircular canal, and jugular bulb.
- The position of the sigmoid sinus is variable. It depends on the degree of mastoid pneumatization.
- Petromastoid canal is open to the posterior cranial fossa through subarcuate cell route (beneath the superior semicircular canal).
- Distance between the vertical facial nerve, sigmoid sinus, and jugular bulb are variable.
- *The Korner's septum* (**Fig. 10**): It extends from the posterior wall of the EAC, it disperses in the air cells close to middle fossa plate, sinodural angle, sigmoid sinus plate, and then runs inferiorly toward the mastoid tip lateral to the facial canal. It is mistaken for the medial wall of the antrum.

Sigmoid Sinus (Fig. 11)

It is continuation of the transverse sinus, passes through the mastoid process in anteroinferior direction to join the jugular bulb (**Flowchart 3**). The posterosuperior part of the sigmoid sinus is the most superior part, inferiorly it passes medial to the digastric ridge and facial nerve to join jugular bulb.
- Most common anatomical variant of the sigmoid sinus is the anterior placement.
- To prevent injury to anterior displaced sigmoid sinus, decompression of the sinus with islets of bone through which one can press down the sinus without injuring it during mastoid surgery.
- Bipolar cauterization makes the sinus shrink.

Sinodural Angle (Citelli's Angle) (Fig. 12)

These cells are situated at the angle between the middle and posterior dura plates. Complete debridement of these cells is required to prevent residual disease.

Posterior Fossa Dural Plate

It separates the mastoid antrum and mastoid air cells from the posterior cranial fossa.

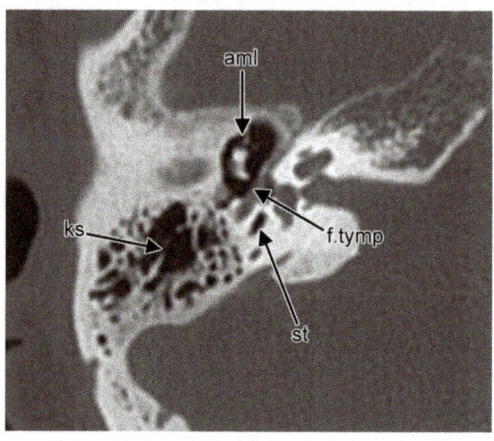

Fig. 11: Computed tomography (CT) scan axial showing the Korner's septum.

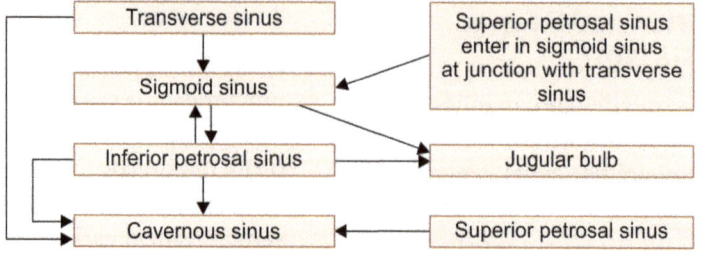

Flowchart 3: The confluence of the various sinuses.

The Trautmann's Triangle

It is an imaginary angle between the labyrinth and middle and posterior cranial fossa dura plate. Through this angle one can assess the posterior cranial fossa from the mastoid antrum.

MASTOID AIR CELL SYSTEM (FLOWCHARTS 4 AND 5)

Computed tomography (CT) scan of the well-pneumatized temporal bone provides an opportunity to describe the distribution of air cells and tracts that compose the mastoid and other pneumatized regions of the temporal bone. These clusters of mucosa lined compartment are ventilated through the aditus ad antrum **(Fig. 13)** or via other cell tracts that open into the middle ear space.

Network of air cells expands along tracts from the middle ear and antrum after third year of life replacing the hemopoietic marrow within the squamous and petrous part of the temporal bone. The mastoid is the largest pneumatized region, lateral to the labyrinth and communicates with attic via its medial compartment, the antrum. The mastoid also extends into occipital bone and communicates with medial cell tract.

Large, pneumatized regions of the mastoid **(Figs. 14A and B)** help in surgical procedure to reach or navigate the deeper structures. An acceptable treatment of chronic otomastoiditis is to exteriorize the poorly aerated mastoid and epitympanum to the EAC.

Defined regions of pneumatization are **(Figs. 15A to D)**:

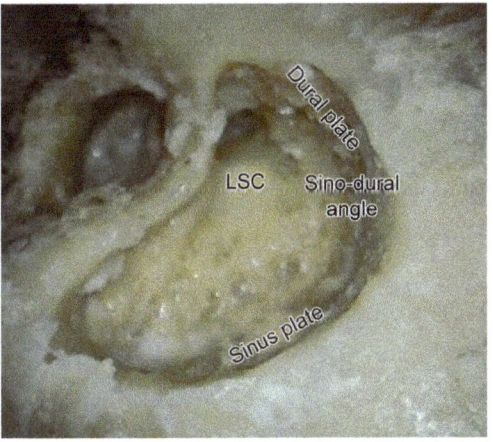

Fig. 12: Cadaveric picture of sinodural angle.

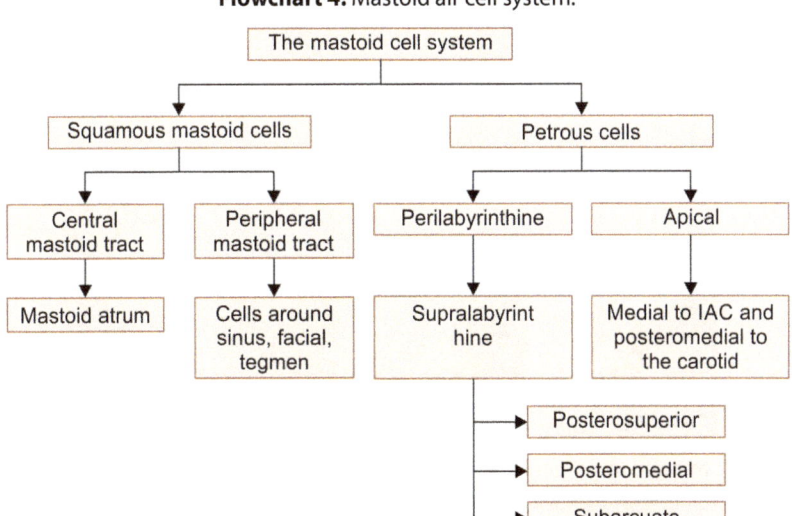

Flowchart 4: Mastoid air cell system.

- *The mastoid:* The central mastoid tract, peripheral mastoid tract (tegmental, sinodural, sinus, facial, and tip cells)
- *Perilabyrinthine cells:* Supralabyrinthine and infralabyrinthine cells
- *The petrous apex:* Peritubal and apical area.

Flowchart 5: The degree of pneumatization.

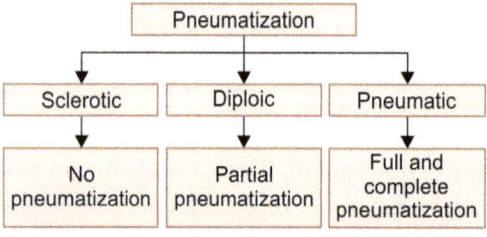

Air cells tracts are paths along which diploic bone and mesenchyme are reabsorbed during maturation, through which air flows to deeper spaces. These tracts circumnavigate the labyrinth and cortical plates of bone that line the middle and posterior fossa dura, sigmoid sinus, carotid artery, and facial nerve. These tracts are also pathways for drainage of spinal fluid to the ear canal or nasopharynx as a result of surgery, trauma, or spontaneous meningoencephalocele.

These pathways are:
- *The posteromedial tract:* It extends from the antrum along the posterior wall of petrous pyramid superior to the internal auditory canal (IAC) toward the apex.
- *The superior tract:* It extends from the epitympanum superior to the labyrinth toward the petrous apex.

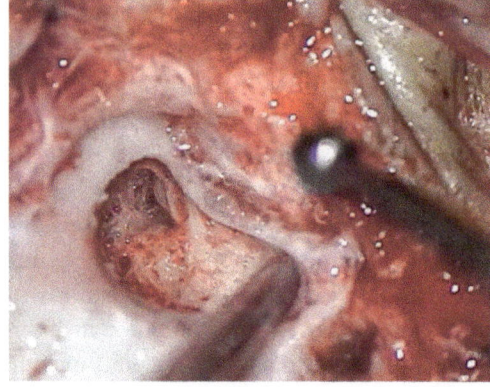

Fig. 13: Microscopic view of aditus ad antrum with the short process of incus and lateral semicircular canal (LSC).

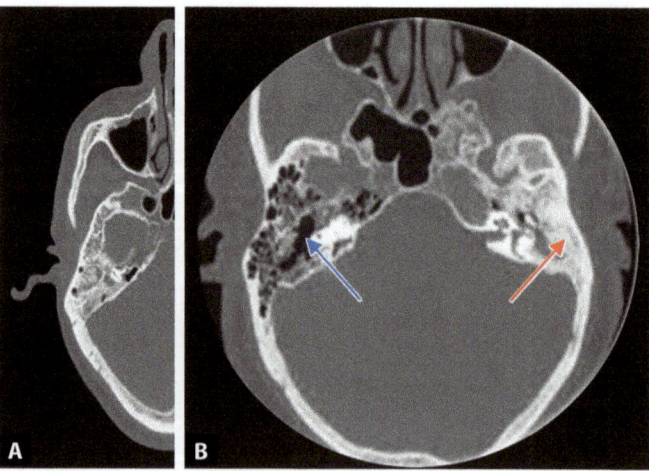

Figs. 14A and B: Computed tomography (CT) of the degrees of pneumatization of the mastoid. [Showing degree of mastoid pneumatization: (A) Diploic mastoid; (B) Pneumatized mastoid on right (blue arrow) and sclerotic mastoid on left (red arrow)].

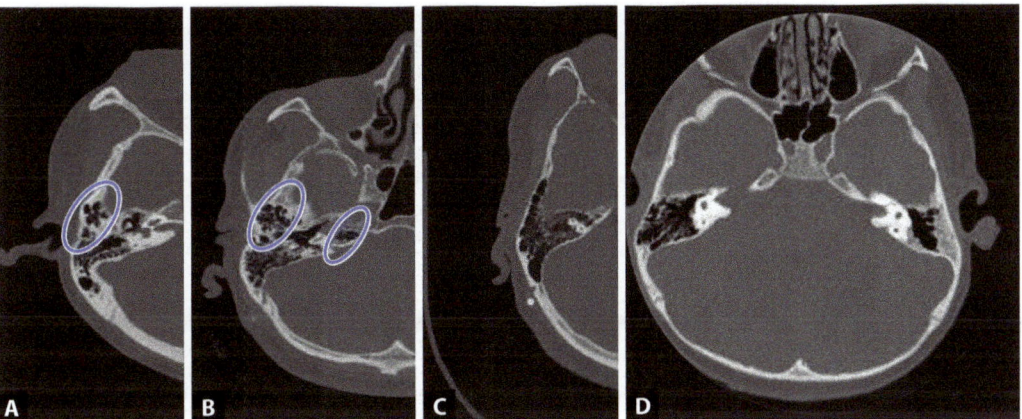

Figs. 15A to D: Different areas of temporal bone pneumatization. [Showing pneumatized mastoid cavity: (A) Mastoid pneumatization with cells also seen in squamous part (Elliptical); (B) Showing pneumatized squamous (large elliptical) and petrous (small elliptical); (C) Well pneumatized mastoid with pneumatized squamosal; (D) Bilateral pneumatized mastoid bone].

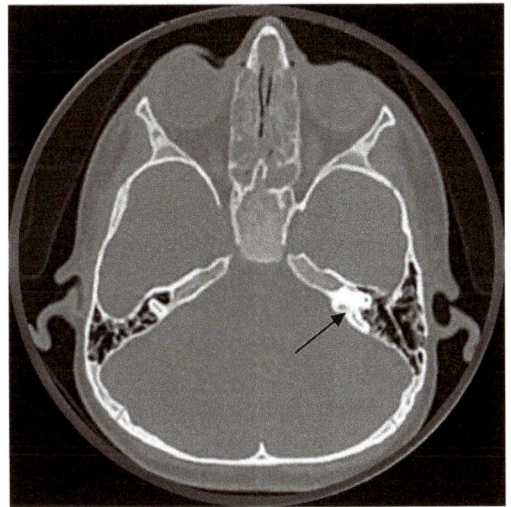

Fig. 16: Subarcuate pathway.

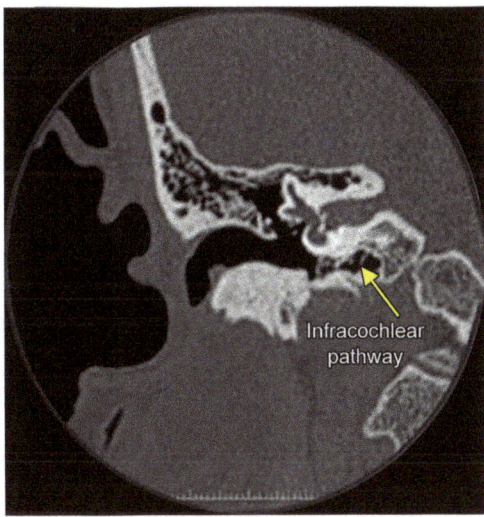

Fig. 17: Inferior tract.

- *Subarcuate tract:* It extends from the antrum to the apex through the center of the superior semicircular canal **(Fig. 16)**.
- *An inferior tract:* It extends from the hypotympanum underneath the cochlea toward the apex **(Fig. 17)**.
- *The anterolateral tract:* That includes the peritubal and pericarotid cells on its course toward the apex.

Drainage of the petrous apex can be achieved by opening cell tracts around the labyrinth through retrolabyrinth, retrofacial, supra, and infralabyrinthine cell tracts **(Figs. 18A and B and 19)**.

Retrofacial dissection is required to reach up to the jugular bulb, posterior petrous apex, and cerebellopontine angle just posterior to the porus acusticus. This is also

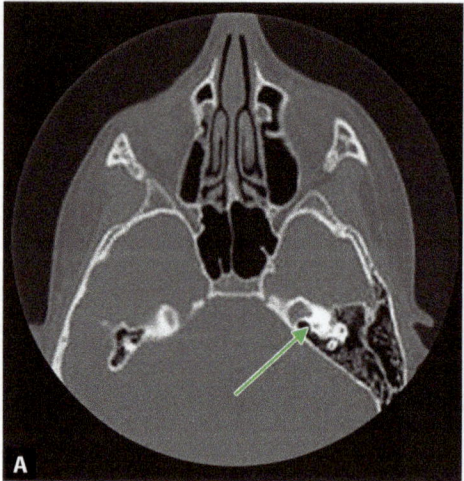 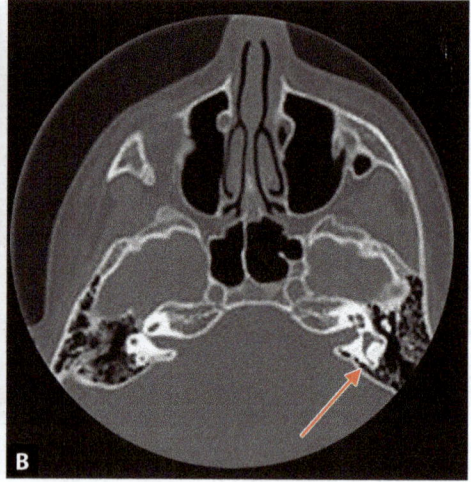

Figs. 18A and B: Perilabyrinthine cell tracts: Supralabyrinthine (green arrow); Infralabyrinthine (red arrow).

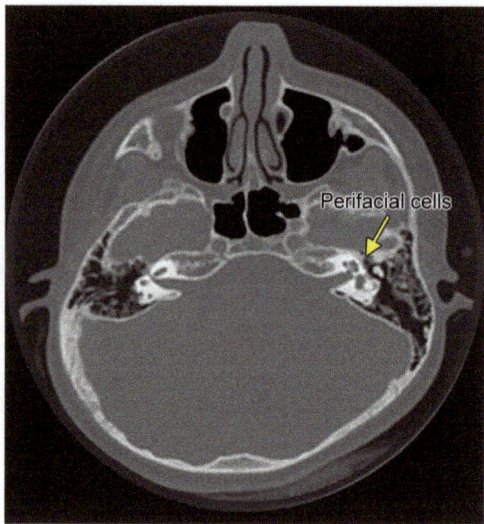

Fig. 19: Perifacial cell.

a common pathway of cerebrospinal fluid (CSF) drainage into the middle ear may occur following surgical decompression of the IAC for removal of a vestibular schwannoma.

BIBLIOGRAPHY

1. Aggarwal R, Saeed SR, Green KJM. Myringoplasty. J Laryngol Otol. 2006;120: 429-32.
2. Anson BDJ. Surgical Anatomy of the Temporal Bone. New York: Raven Press; 1992.
3. Atmaca S, Elmali M, Kucuk H. High and dehiscent jugular bulb: clear and present danger during middle ear surgery. Surg Radiol Anat. 2014;36:369-74.
4. Eby TL. Development of the facial recess: implications for cochlear implantation. Laryngoscope. 1996;106 (5 Pt 2 Suppl 80): 1-7.
5. Friedmann DR, Eubig J, McGill M, Babb JS, Pramanik BK, Lalwani AK. Development of the jugular bulb: a radiologic study. Otol Neurotol. 2011;32(8):1389-95.
6. Friedmann DR, Le BT, Pramanik BK, Lalwani AK. Clinical spectrum of patients with erosion of the inner ear by jugular bulb abnormalities. Laryngoscope. 2010;120(2):365-72.
7. Graham MD. The jugular bulb: its anatomic and clinical considerations in contemporary otology. Laryngoscope. 1977;87(1):105-25.
8. Lim DJ. Tympanic membrane: electron microscopic observations, part II: pars fláccida. Acta Otolaryngol. 1968;66: 515-32.
9. Miklós Tóth, Pre- and postnatal changes in the human tympanic cavity, Semmelweis University School of Doctoral Studies

for Developmental Biology Ph.D. Thesis, Budapest; 2007.
10. Roland Jr JT, Hoffman RA, Miller PJ, Cohen NL. Retrofacial approach to the hypotympanum. Arch Otolaryngol Head Neck Surg. 1995;121(2):233-6.
11. Sadé J. Retraction pockets and attic cholesteatomas. Acta Otorhinolaryngol Belg. 1980;34:62-84.
12. Sanna M, Fois P, Paolo F, Russo A, Falcioni M. Management of meningoencephalic herniation of the temporal bone: personal experience and literature review. Laryngoscope. 2009;119:1579-85.
13. Spector GJ, Ge XX. Development of the hypotympanum in the human fetus and neonate. Ann Otol Rhinol Laryngol Suppl. 1981;90(6 Pt 2):1-20.

CHAPTER 4

Facial Nerve

INTRODUCTION

Facial nerve **(Fig. 1)** is the nerve of facial expression. Its dysfunction gives remarkable disfigurement and emotional stress as it affects "nonverbal humanistic expression". Facial nerve paralysis affects normal daily functions such as eating, drinking, and loss of protective function of eye. The understanding of complex anatomy of the facial nerve is essential to diagnose and treat the facial nerve dysfunction.

FACIAL NERVE DEVELOPMENT (FIG. 2)

At about 3rd week of gestation, facial nerve appears as facioacoustic primordium (arising from rhombencephalon) which impinges on deep aspect of the second branchial arch. Facial nerve, motor division arises in the embryonic pons and sensory division arises from the cranial neural crest. At around 4th week, first branch, chorda tympani appear, approximately same size as the facial nerve. Around 5th week of gestation, sensory part becomes evident as independent nerve. The chorda tympani and the lingual nerve unite just near to the ganglion. The greater superficial petrosal nerve which arises from the anterior aspect of the geniculate ganglion appears in same time.

At around 8th week, cartilaginous capsule from the ear vesicles forms a groove around the facial nerve, stapedial artery and

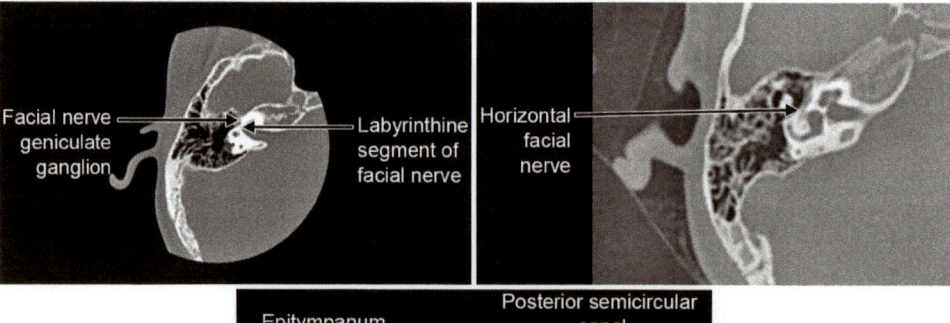
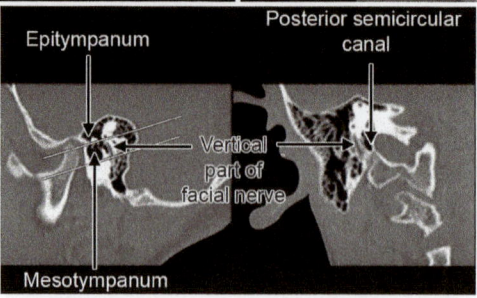

Fig. 1: High-resolution computed tomography temporal bone with radiology of facial nerve.

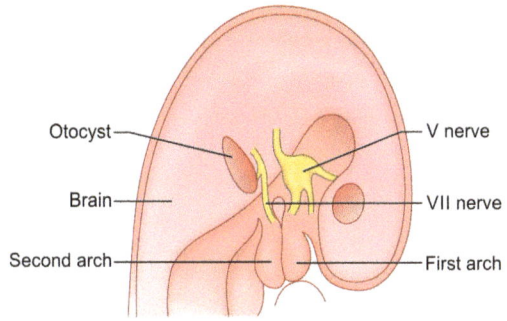

Fig. 2: Embryology of facial nerve.

stapedius muscle, eventually develops into facial canal.

At around 12th week, all muscles of the face develop, which are innervated by a branch of the facial nerve.

At 7th week, a ventral offshoot from the geniculate ganglion toward the glossopharyngeal ganglion forms the tympanic plexus and the lesser petrosal nerve. At the same time, nerve to stapedius muscle arises. Between the 12th and 13th weeks, two twigs between the stapedius and the chorda tympani fuse and extend to the 9th and 10th cranial nerve and form the Arnold's nerve.

By 17th week, definitive communications of facial nerve with 5th nerve, 9th nerve, 10th nerve, and 2nd and 3rd cervical nerves are established.

Trajectory of the facial nerve in intrauterine life: Facial nerve—at first is rectilinear structure, at 6th week due to mesencephalic growth, change of direction occurs in acute angle and at 4th month, another change in direction occurs secondary to the development of the tympanic cavity.

Ossification of the cartilaginous otic capsule (facial canal): There are two ossification centers, anterior one at the apical cochlear ossification and a posterior one arising at pyramidal eminence. Complete development occurs at around 3 months after birth.

ANATOMY (FIG. 3)

The facial nerve is the nerve of second branchial arch, mixed nerve containing motor sensory and secretomotor components. It is composed of 10,000 neurons; majority 7,000 myelinated neurons form the motor part, and the 3,000 neurons form the nervous intermedius.

The facial nerve has four nuclei (**Flowchart 1**):
1. Branchiomotor nucleus
2. Superior salivatory nucleus
3. Lacrimatory nucleus
4. Nucleus of tractus solitarius.

The path of the facial nerve can be divided into six segments:
1. Intracranial (cisternal) segment
2. Meatal (canalicular) segment [within internal auditory canal (IAC)]
3. Labyrinthine segment (IAC to the geniculate ganglion)
4. Tympanic segment (from geniculate ganglion to the pyramidal eminence)
5. Mastoid segment (from pyramidal eminence to stylomastoid foramen)
6. Extratemporal segment.

The facial nerve innervates structures derived from Reichert's cartilage (muscles of facial expression, stapedius muscle, stylohyoid and posterior belly of the digastric), the superior aspect of the motor nucleus, innervating the frontalis and orbicularis oculi muscles, receives both crossed and uncrossed input from the motor center, while inferior portion receives only ipsilateral input.

The facial nerve (**Fig. 4**) exits the pontomedullary junction, caudal to the trigeminal nerve and it is approximately 1.5 mm anterior, superior, and medial to the vestibulocochlear nerve (size of facial nerve is smaller diameter than the 8th nerve 1.8 mm versus 3 mm). The facial nerve, nervus intermedius, and the vestibulocochlear nerves are crossing the

46 Facial Nerve

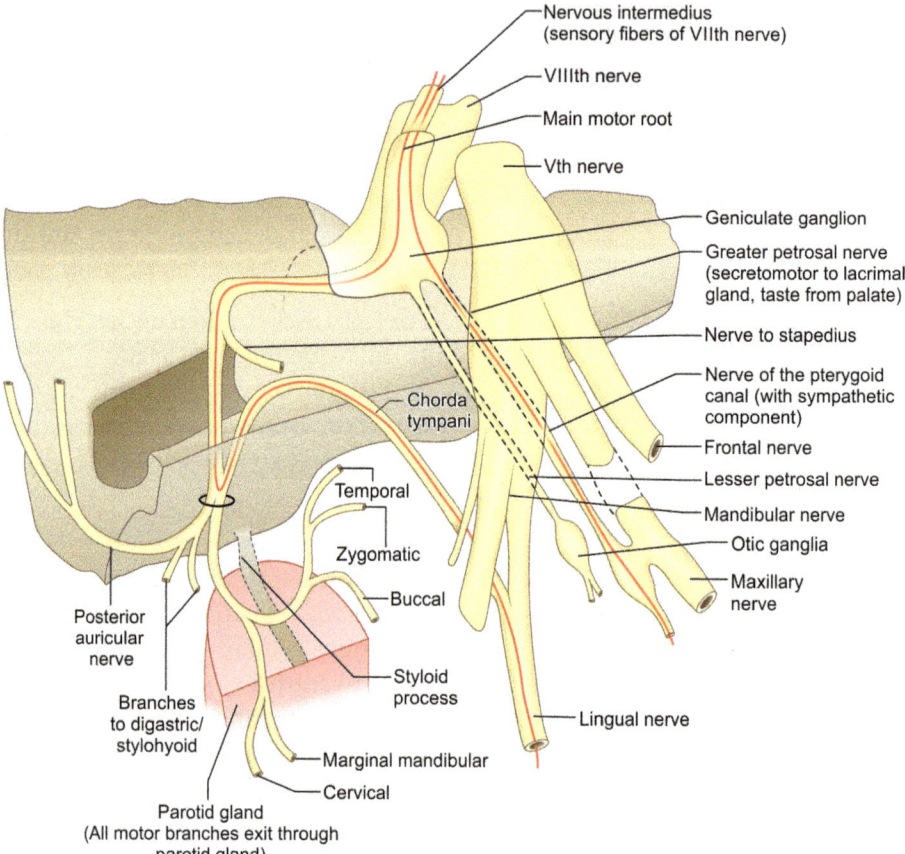

Fig. 3: Facial nerve branches.

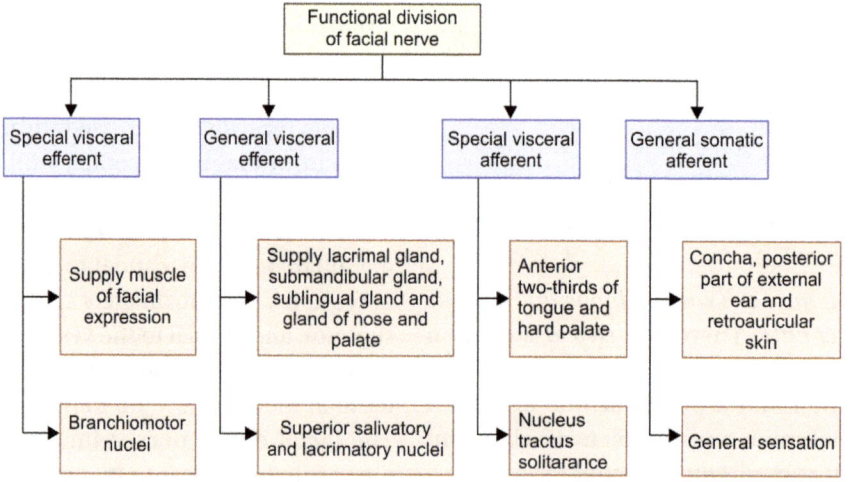

Flowchart 1: The nuclei of the facial nerve.

Facial Nerve

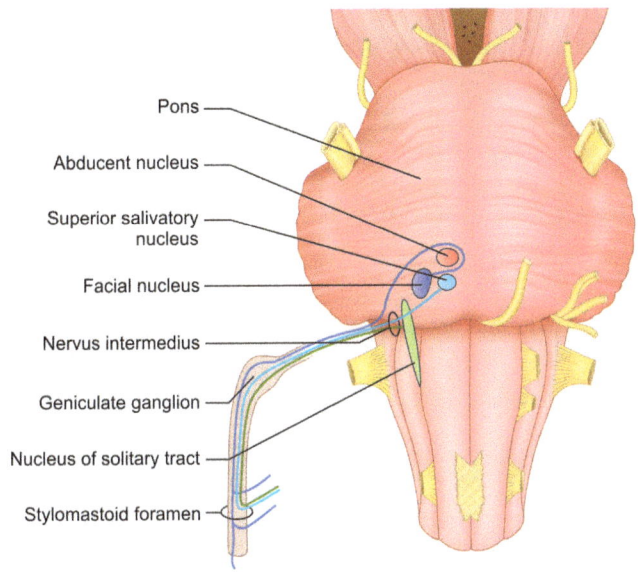

Fig. 4: The intracranial course of the facial nerve.

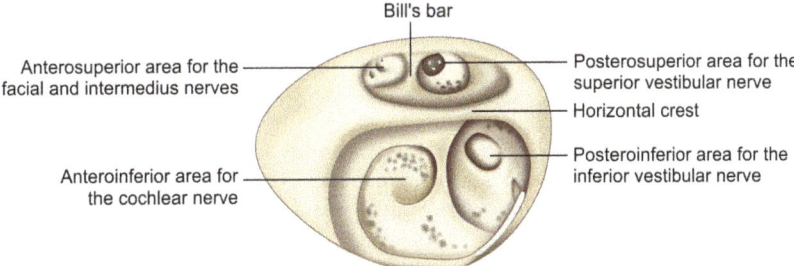

Fig. 5: The internal auditory meatus cross-section view, depicting Bill's bar.

cerebellopontine angle (15-17 mm distance) and enters the IAC.

In the internal auditory meatus (around 8-10 mm length), facial nerve **(Fig. 5)** is anterior and superior, and inferior vestibulocochlear nerve lies immediately posterior and posteroinferior to the facial nerve.

The cochlear nerve lies inferior to the facial nerve in the IAC. When the facial nerve reaches up to the fundus, it merges with the sensory component (nervus intermedius).

Then labyrinthine segment of the facial nerve **(Fig. 6)** starts as it enters the meatal foramen, which is the narrowest part of the canal, adjacent to the canal dense arachnoid band, encircles the nerve give rise to "bottle neck," anatomical site that can constrict the nerve in response to edema. Labyrinthine segment is bounded anteriorly by the cochlea, posteriorly by the superior semicircular canal, inferiorly the vestibule, and superiorly the middle cranial fossa.

Subsequently fallopian canal provides a bony covering to the nerve, it takes long, tortuous pathway through the temporal bone.

At the geniculate ganglion, nerve takes sharp posterior turn (60-90°) at the first genu. Geniculate ganglion contains bipolar

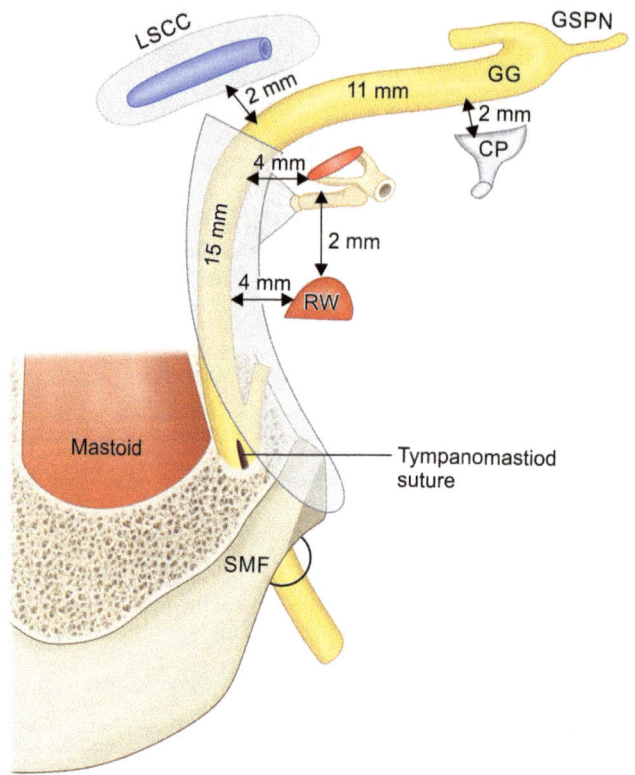

Fig. 6: Tympanomastoid segment of the facial nerve and its relations with middle ear structures. (CP: cochleariformis process; GG: geniculate ganglion; LSCC: lateral semicircular canal; GSPN: greater superficial petrosal nerve; RW: round window; SMF: stylomastoid foramen)

ganglion cells for the sensory part of the facial nerve. The greater superficial petrosal nerve arises from the anterior aspect of the geniculate ganglion, and it passes through facial hiatus at the middle cranial fossa, joins the deep petrosal nerve. From the pterygopalatine ganglion it gives rise to secretory fibers to the lacrimal gland.

The tympanic segment of the facial nerve **(Fig. 6)** (11–13 mm) runs obliquely posteriorly from superior aspect of the supratubal recess up to the superior aspect of the oval window, then posterior to the oval window, it takes turn from the medial wall of tympanic cavity to the posterior wall of the tympanic cavity, forms the vertical or mastoid part of the facial nerve (13 mm). Here, it turns and forms the second genu of the facial nerve, nerve is anteroinferior to the horizontal semicircular canal, medial to the short process of incus and posterolateral to the pyramidal eminence.

Approximately midway in this segment, the chorda tympani nerve and nerve to stapedius muscle arise (between the second genu and stylomastoid foramen).

Facial nerve gives parasympathetic fibers to the sublingual and submandibular gland (chorda tympani nerve) to the lacrimal gland **(Fig. 7)** (pterygopalatine ganglion). The facial nerve leaves the temporal bone through stylomastoid foramen lying between the stylomastoid foramen lying between

Facial Nerve

the mastoid tip and the styloid process. At foramen, it is encircled by the digastric muscle fibrous tendon. Sharp, meticulous dissection is required to release the nerve.

In parotid gland, extratemporal part divides into the temporofacial and cervicofacial trunks. Each nerve fiber has nerve cell body and axon surrounded by layer of myelin secreted by Schwann cells. A single nerve fiber is surrounded by multiple Schwann cells. Each nerve fiber is surrounded by the connective tissue layers, endoneurium forms the tubule. Multiple tubules surrounded by perineurium. Additional neural sheath forms the epineurium. These three connective tissues (endoneurium, perineurium, and epineurium)

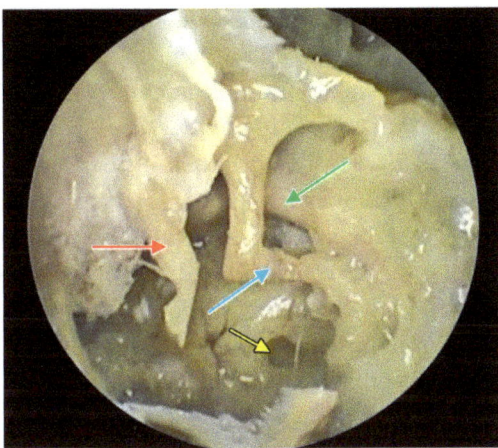

Fig. 7: Endoscopic cadaveric view of tympanic segment of the facial nerve. [Tympanic segment of facial nerve (green arrow); round window (yellow arrow); malleus (red arrow); IS joint (blue arrow)].

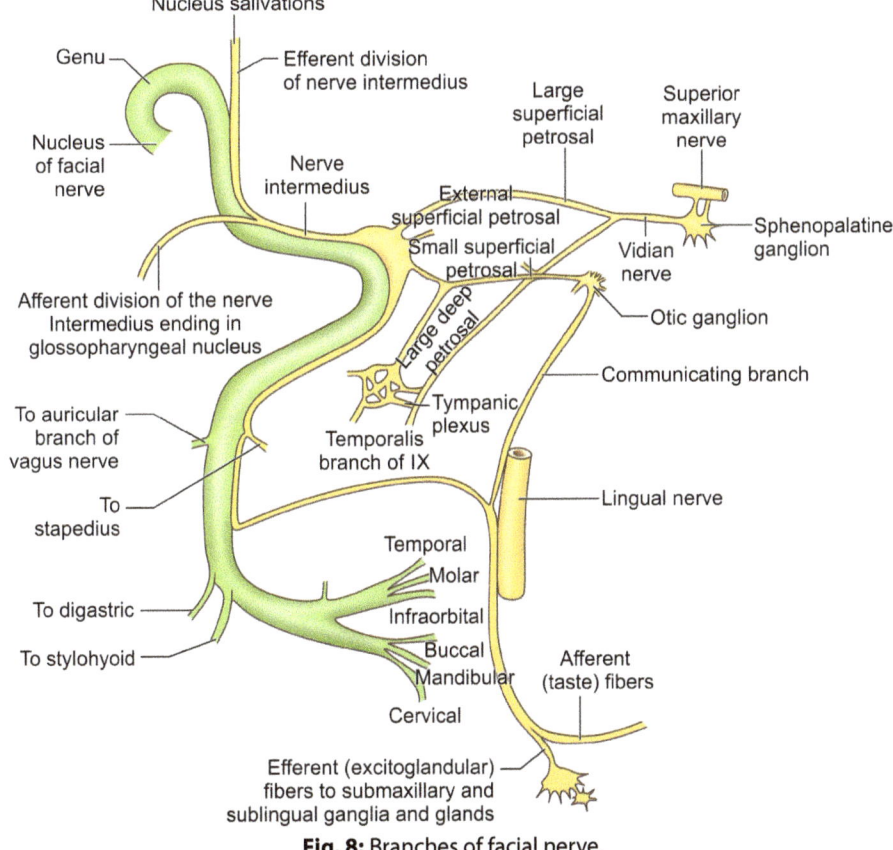

Fig. 8: Branches of facial nerve.

play important functions including resisting stretching, maintaining tensile strength and intraneural pressures. All the branches of facial nerve is well illustrated in the figure above **(Fig. 8)**

ANOMALIES OF THE FACIAL NERVE (FIGS. 9A TO G)

- *Internal auditory meatus:* Variation in depth of the internal auditory meatus (at both ends) affects the width of facial nerve.
- *Labyrinthine segment:* It shows variable distance between the geniculate ganglion and the labyrinthine segment.
- *In the tympanic cavity:* Displacement of nerve, dehiscence, bifurcation, or trifurcation of nerve.

The facial nerve may displace, at or inferior to the oval window, between the oval window and the round window.

Developmental variations of the labyrinth also affect the facial nerve.

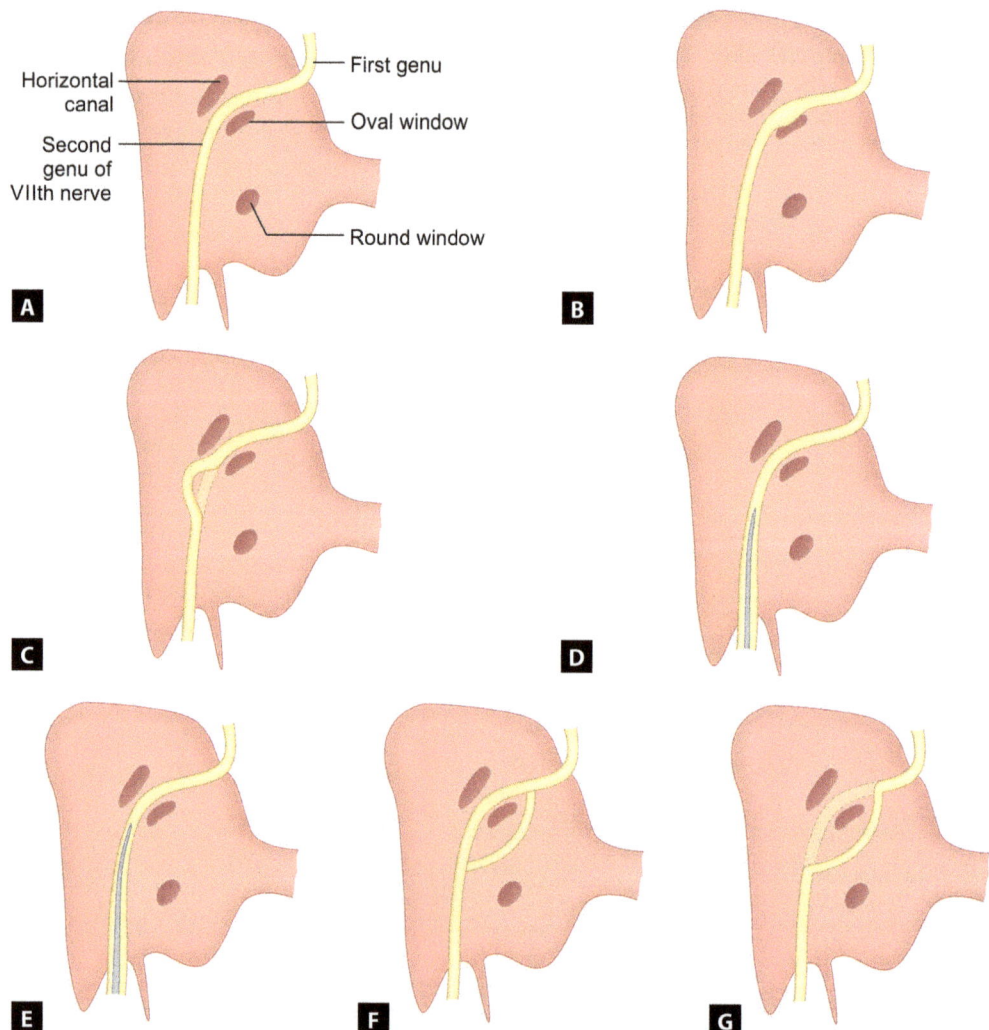

Figs. 9A to G: Variations of the facial nerve in the middle ear.

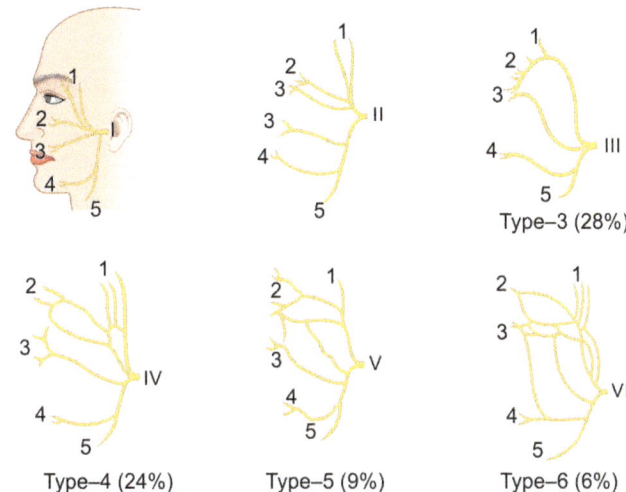

Fig. 10: Variation of facial nerve branching in the parotid.
(1: Temporal/frontal; 2: Zygomatic; 3: Buccal; 4: Mandibular; 5: Cervical)

Anatomical variations of facial nerve are also seen within parotid **(Fig. 10)**.

Vascular Supply (Fig. 11)

Main arterial supply of the facial nerve is:
- The labyrinthine artery—a branch of anterior inferior cerebellar artery
- The superior petrosal artery—a branch of middle meningeal artery
- The stylomastoid artery—a branch of postauricular artery.

These three branches constitute the extrinsic vascular system. The intraneural vascular plexus (intrinsic system) originates from the extrinsic system.

■ SURGICAL ANATOMY

As the mastoid process is not developed till 1 year of age, the facial nerve exits through the stylomastoid foramen which lies to lateral aspect of the skull, this makes the facial nerve vulnerable to the surgical or the traumatic injury.

Abnormal development of the tympanic bone leads to the displacement of the mastoid segment of facial nerve posteriorly. The common anomaly of the facial nerve is anterior displacement.

Hemifacial spasm occurs due to vascular compression at the root exit zone.

The subarachnoid space of the facial nerve usually extends up to the labyrinthine segment of the facial nerve, occasionally it extends to the geniculate ganglion or rarely up to the lateral aspect of the tympanic segment may lead to spontaneous cerebrospinal fluid (CSF) otorrhea.

In Gusher syndrome, which is an X-linked congenital mixed deafness, there is a communication between high pressure CSF in IAC and perilymph of inner ear leads to leakage, causing the stapes gusher during stapes surgery.

The greater superficial petrosal nerve is the essential landmark during the middle cranial fossa surgery.

The section of greater superficial petrosal nerve (GSPN) or vidian nerve is vital for vasomotor rhinitis.

Second genu of the facial nerve is the most common site for the iatrogenic injury

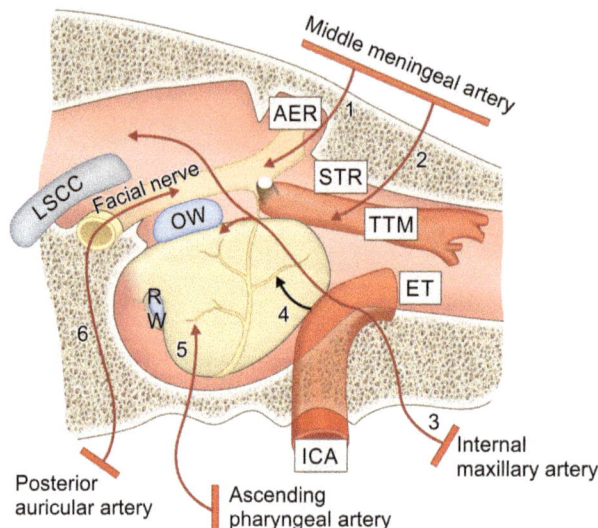

Fig. 11: Vasculature of the facial nerve. (AER: anterior epitympanic recess; ET: Eustachian tube; ICA: internal carotid artery; LSCC: lateral semicircular canal; OW: oval window; RW: round window; STR: supratubal recess; TTM: tensor tympani muscle; 1: Superficial petrosal artery; 2: Superior tympanic artery; 3: Anterior tympanic artery; 4: Caroticotympanic artery; 5: Inferior tympanic artery; 6: Stylomastoid artery)

during ear surgery (in case of invasive cholesteatoma).

The facial recess approach is dynamic approach for the structures of the retrotympanum (transmastoid).

Facial recess **(Fig. 12)** boundaries are:
- *Posterolaterally:* Mastoid segment of facial nerve
- *Anteromedially:* Medially chorda tympani nerve
- *Superiorly:* Incudal buttress.

The facial nerve exits through stylomastoid foramen, it lies anteromedial to digastric ridge. The sigmoid sinus lies posteromedial to the facial nerve.

The "cog" and the cochleariformis process is important landmark for the tympanic segment of facial nerve.

The tympanic annulus should not be considered a secure landmark for identification of facial nerve during canaloplasty.

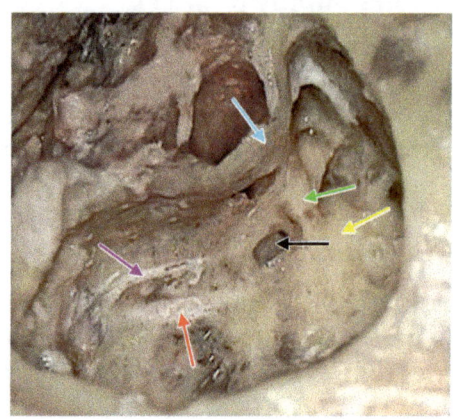

Fig. 12: Cadaveric view of the facial recess. [Posterior EAC (blue arrow); incus buttress (green arrow); LSC (yellow arrow); chordatympani (purple arrow); vertical facial nerve (red arrow); facial recess (black arrow)].

During cortical mastoidectomy:
- Crucial landmarks for the identification of facial nerve in the mastoid cavity are:
  - Horizontal semicircular canal

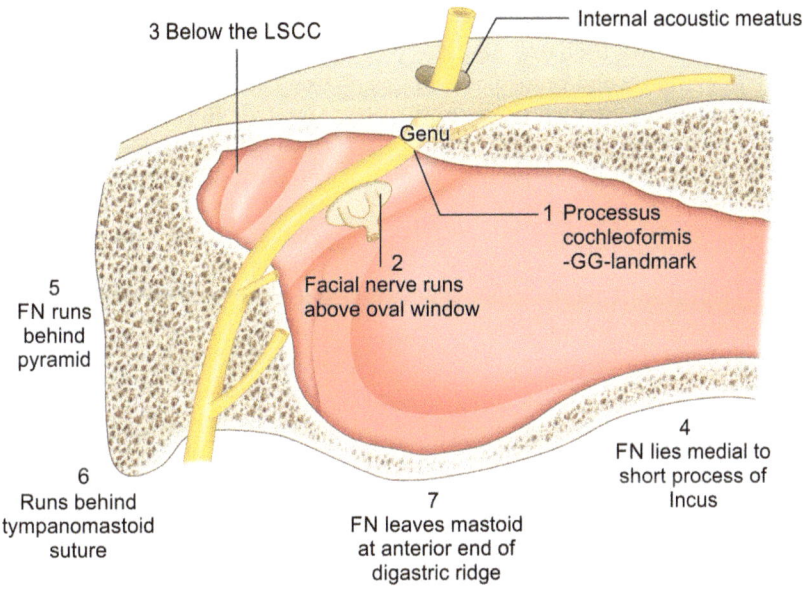

Fig. 13: Surgical landmarks of the facial nerve.

- Short process of incus
- Mastoid tip.

The facial nerve lies anteroinferior to the lateral semicircular canal (LSC), then it travels inferiorly toward the digastric ridge. The bone of the EAC is progressively thinned into a direction parallel to the nerve, until the white sheath is identified through bone.

In lateral skull base surgery, rerouting of the facial nerve reduces the blood supply of the facial nerve with high risk of facial weakness.

Surgical landmarks of the facial nerve in middle ear cleft are **(Fig. 13)**:
- Processus cochleariformis
- Cog
- Oval window
- Horizontal semicircular canal
- Short process of incus
- Pyramid
- Tympanomastoid suture
- Digastric ridge.

Parotid gland surgery:
- *Tragal cartilage pointer:* It is a sharp triangular extension of the tragal cartilage which points toward the facial nerve. The facial nerve lies 1–1.5 cm inferior and medially
- Styloid process
- Posterior belly of digastric
- *Mastoid process:* It follows the anterior border of the mastoid process up to the vaginal process of the tympanic bone. It bisects the tympanomastoid angle at the tympanomastoid suture.

BIBLIOGRAPHY

1. Adad B, Rasgon BM, Ackerson L. Relationship of the facial nerve to the tympanic annulus: a direct anatomic examination. Laryngoscope. 1999;109(8):1189-92.
2. Badr-El-Dine M, El-Garem HF, Talaat AM, Magnan J. Endoscopically assisted minimally invasive microvascular decompression

of hemifacial spasm. Otol Neurotol. 2002;23(2):122-8.
3. Bast TH, Anson BJ, Richany SF. The development of the second branchial arch (Reichert's cartilage), facial canal and associated structures in man. Q Bull Northwest Univ Med Sch. 1956;30:235-49.
4. Baxter A. Dehiscence of the fallopian canal. An anatomical study. J Laryngol Otol. 1971; 85(6):587-94.
5. Chandra S, Goyal M, Gandhi D, Gera S, Berry M. Anatomy of the facial nerve in the temporal bone: HRCT. Indian J Radiol Imaging. 1999;9(1):5-8.
6. Chi FL, Wang J, Yuan YS, Liu HJ, Gu J, Huang T, et al. Landmark of facial nerve in middle ear surgery. Zhonghua Er Bi Yan Hou Tou Jing Wai Ke Za Zhi. 2006;41(1):5-8.
7. Clark MP, O'Malley S. Chorda tympani nerve function after middle ear surgery. Otol Neurotol. 2007;28(3):335-40.
8. Cornelia U (Ed). Paralizii le nervu lui facial. Laşi: Ars Longa; 2001. pp. 11-7.
9. Gantz Bruce J, Rubinstein Jay T. Intratemporal facial nerve surgery. In: CW Cummings, JM Fredrickson, LA Harker, CJ Krause, MA Richardson, DE Schuller (Eds). Otolaryngology Head and Neck Surgery, 3rd edition, Volume 4, Issue 143. St. Louis: Mosby—Year Book, Inc.; 1998;4(143): pp. 2785-99.
10. Ge XX, Spector GJ. Labyrinthine segment and geniculate ganglion of the facial nerve in fetal and adult temporal bones. Ann Otol Rhinol Laryngol. 1981;90 (Suppl 85):1-12.
11. Gopalan P, Kumar M, Gupta D, Phillips JJ. A study of chorda tympani nerve injury and related symptoms following middle-ear surgery. J Laryngol Otol. 2005;119(3):189-92.
12. GulyaIn AJ. Developmental anatomy of the temporal bone and skull base. In: Glasscock-Shambaugh's Surgery of the Ear, 6th edition. Shelton: People's Medical Publishing House; 2010. pp. 3-27.
13. Hofmann L. Der Faserverlauf im N. facialis. Z Hals Nas Ohrenheilk. 1924;10:86.
14. Jongkees LBW. Die chirurgische Behandlung der intrtemporalen Facialishahmung. Dtsch Med Wochenschr. 1958;83:865.
15. Joseph MP, Guinan Jr JJ, Fullerton BC, Norris BE, Kiang NY. Number and distribution of stapedius motoneurons in cats. J Comp Neurol. 1985;232:43-54.
16. Kim CW, Rho YS, Ahn HY, Oh SJ. Facial canal dehiscence in the initial operation for chronic otitis media without cholesteatoma. Auris Nasus Larynx. 2008;35(3):353-6.
17. Kiverniti E, Watters G. Taste disturbance after mastoid surgery: immediate and long-term effects of chorda tympani nerve sacrifice. J Laryngol Otol. 2012;126(1):34-7.
18. Kumar G, Castello M, Bucman CA. X-linked stapes gusher; CT findings in one patient. Am J Neuroradiol. 2003;24:1130-2.
19. Lindemann H. The fallopian canal. An anatomical study of its distal part. Acta Otolaryngol Suppl. 1960;158:204.
20. Louryan S. Développement du nerf facial. In: Martin- Duverneuil N (Ed). A propos du nerf facial. Paris: Guerbet; 1994. pp. 3-9.
21. Lyon MJ. The central location of the motor neurons to the stapedius muscle in the cat. Brain Res. 1978;143(3):437-44.
22. Magnan J, Caces F, Locatelli P, Chays A. Hemifacial spasm: endoscopic vascular decompression. Otolaryngol Head Neck Surg. 1997;117(4):308-14.
23. Magnan J, Chays A, Caces F, Lepetre-Gillot C, Cohen JM, Belus JF, et al. Role of endoscopy and vascular decompression in the treatment of hemifacial spasm. Ann Otolaryngol Chir Cervicofac. 1994;111(3):153-60.
24. Magnan J, Chays A. Functional surgery on the acoustic-facial pedicle. Rev Laryngol Otol Rhinol (Bord). 1998;119(3):151-4.
25. Mahendran S, Hogg R, Robinson JM. To divide or manipulate the chorda tympani in stapedotomy. Eur Arch Otorhinolaryngol. 2005;262(6):482-7.
26. Miehlke A. Uber die Topographie des Faserverlaufes im Facialisstamm. Arch Ohren Nasen Kehlkopfheilkd. 1958;171:340.
27. Măru N, Cheiţă AC, Mogoantă CA, Prejoianu B. Intratemporal course of the facial nerve: morphological, topographic and morphometric features. Rom J Morphol Embryol. 2010;51(2):243-8.

28. Măru N, Cheiță AC, Mogoantă CA, Prejoianu B. Intratemporal course of the facial nerve: morphological, topographic and morphometric features. Rom J Morphol Embryol. 2010;51(2):243-8.
29. Ozgirgin N, Cenjor C, Filipo R, Magnan J. Consensus on treatment algorithms for traumatic and iatrogenic facial paralysis. Mediterr J Otol. 2007;3:150-8.
30. Pellet W, Cannoni M, Pech A. Basic anatomy. In: Otoneurosurgery. Berlin: Springer; 1990. pp. 5-72.
31. Proctor B. Surgical anatomy of the ear and temporal bone. New York: Thieme Medical Publishers; 1989.
32. Spector JG, Ge X. Ossification patterns of the tympanic facial canal in the human fetus and neonate. Laryngoscope. 1993;103:1052-65.
33. Talbot JM, Wilson DF. Computed tomographic diagnosis of X-linked congenital mixed deafness, fixation of the stapedial footplate, and perilymphatic gusher. Am J Otol. 1994;15(2):177-82.
34. Tóth M, Moser G, Patonay L, Oláh I. Development of the anterior chordal canal. Ann Anat. 2006;188(1):7-11.
35. Wetmore RF, Muntz HR, McGill TJ. Pediatric Otolaryngology: Principles and Practice Pathways. New York: Thieme Medical Publishers; 2000.
36. Yadav S, Ranga A, Sirohiwal B. Surgical anatomy of tympano-mastoid segment of facial nerve. Indian J Otolaryngol Head Neck Surg. 2006;58(1):27-30.
37. Yamakami I, Uchino Y, Kobayashi E, Yamaura A. Computed tomography evaluation of air cells in the petrous bone–relationship with postoperative cerebrospinal fluid rhinorrhea. Neurol Med Chir (Tokyo). 2003;43(7):334-8; discussion.

Eustachian Tube

THE EUSTACHIAN TUBE

It is a fibrocartilaginous tube extending from the (tympani orifice) anterior wall of the middle ear cavity to the nasopharynx. The pharyngotympanic tube develops from the tubotympanic recess. Constriction of this recess forms the primordial Eustachian tube medially and primordial tympanic cavity laterally.

It is around 36 mm in length. It develops remarkably in early years of life. It has a bony and cartilaginous part.

Anatomy of Eustachian Tube (Fig. 1)

Bony Part

The bony part is around 12 mm of length which extends from the tympani orifice in the protympanum to the junction of the squamous and petrous bone with irregular and uneven edge. The tympanic orifice is wide and it relates to the cochlea, internal carotid artery, tensor tympani canal, and bony septum separating the tensor tympani muscle **(Fig. 2)**. Its superior wall is called tegmen tuberi. The width of the bony part is decreased as it goes toward the junctional part (cartilage part). Junctional part is the narrowest part of the Eustachian tube and it called "isthmus." The isthmus is narrow part lies between the internal carotid artery medially, foramen spinosum, and the middle meningeal artery laterally.

The fibrocartilaginous part: It extends from the nasopharynx to the isthmus around 24 mm in length. It lies in the inferior aspect of the skull at the junction of the greater wing of sphenoid with petrous apex bone in "sulcus tubae" (groove) and it enters the lateral wall of nasopharynx by piercing the buccopharyngeal fascia and pharyngobasilar fascia at sinus Morgagni (Base skull) above the superior constrictor muscle.

Direction of the Eustachian tube is downward, forward, and medially toward the nasopharynx. Bony and cartilaginous parts of the Eustachian tube are not in the same plane. Eustachian tube is tightly fixed at tubercle on the posterior edge of the medial pterygoid plate.

At nasopharynx, lumen is the widest and it is around the same level as the inferior nasal concha. Tubal elevation around the

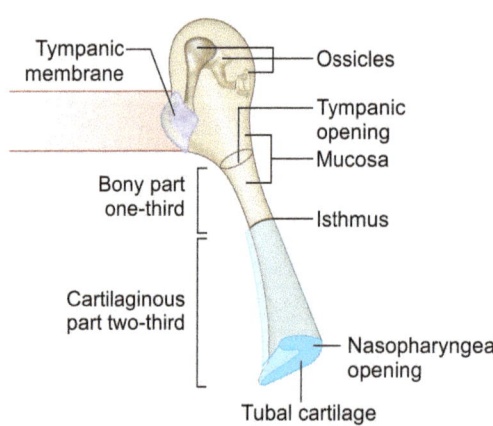

Fig. 1: Eustachian tube anatomy horizontal section.

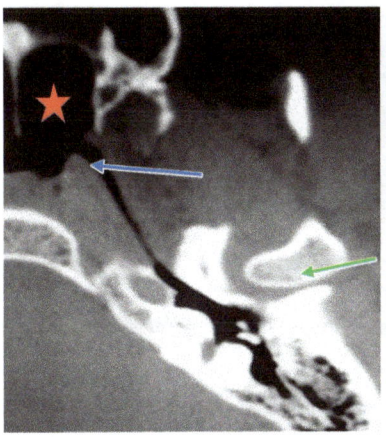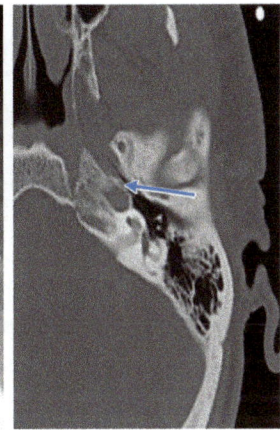

Fig. 2: Computed tomography (CT) scan showing Eustachian tube. [Eustachian tube as seen in axial section of HRCT temporal bone. Nasopharynx (red star); eustachian tube (blue arrow); temporomandibular joint (green arrow)].

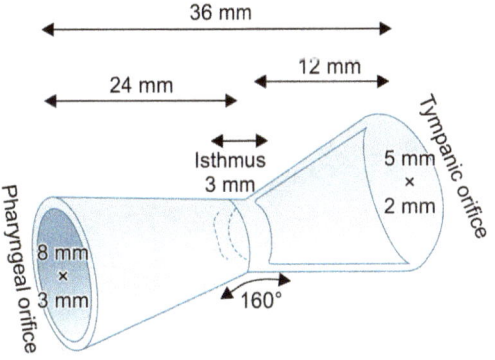

Fig. 3: Dimensions of Eustachian tube.

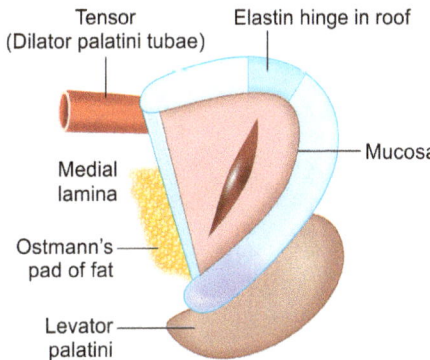

Fig. 4: Ostmann's pad of fat.

Eustachian tube is due to submucous coat of lymphoid tissue (tubal tonsil) **(Fig. 3)**.

The cartilaginous portion of tube is composed of "J"-shaped cartilage (broad medial, small lateral lamina) and fibrous tube or connective tissue is occupied in the lateral and inferior wall of fibrocartilaginous tube. The base of cartilage produces tubal elevation at the nasopharynx and apex of it connected to the bony part of the Eustachian tube.

Ostmann's pad of fat **(Fig. 4)** is basically lymphoadipose tissue around the inferolateral aspect of the anterior part of the Eustachian tube. It occupies between the Eustachian tube and tensor veli palatini muscle. Eustachian tube prevents the secretion or regurgitation of fluid from pharynx to the ear. In malnourished patient, this fat is lost causing and patulous Eustachian tube.

Muscles associate with the Eustachian tube **(Fig. 5)**:
- Levator veli palatini
- Tensor tympani
- Tensor veli palatini
- Salpingopharyngeus.

The tube remains close at rest. Tensor veli palatini contraction causes active opening of the tube, closing phenomenon is passive **(Figs. 6A and B)**.

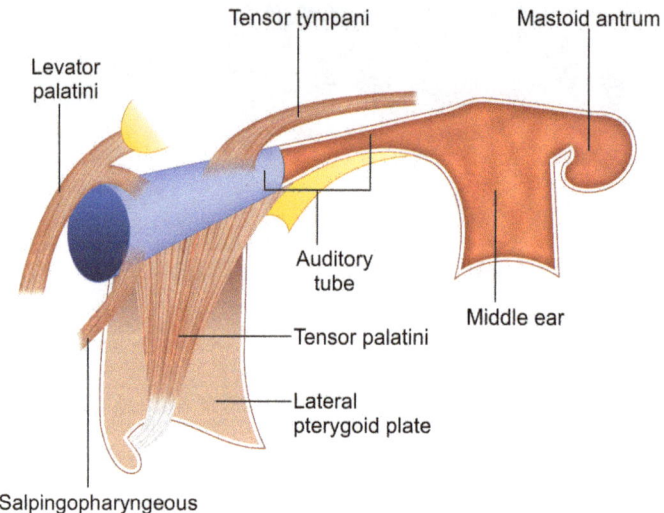

Fig. 5: Eustachian tube muscles.

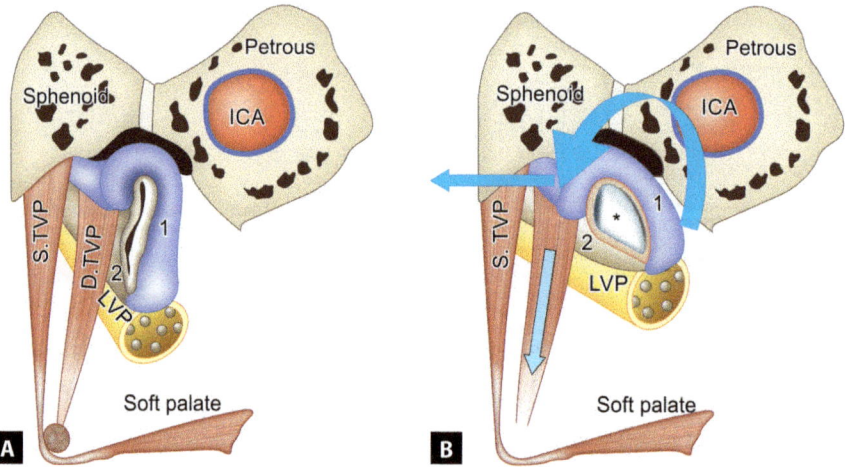

Figs. 6A and B: Paratubal muscles and action of tensor veli palatine. (A) During relaxation and (B) during contraction. (ICA: internal carotid artery; LVP: levator veli palatine muscle; S. TVP: superficial bundle of tensor veli palatine muscle; L: tubal ligament; 1: tubal cartilage; 2: tubal fibrous membrane; *: tubal lumen; H: hamulus)

Mucosal Lining of Eustachian Tube

The cartilaginous part of the Eustachian tube is lined with a ciliated columnar epithelium and toward tympanic orifice are nonciliated and flat cuboidal cells with less goblet cells. The Eustachian tube is having superior corridor for the gaseous exchange (ventilation) and inferior corridor (floor) is for mucociliary function.

The Eustachian tube supplied by the ascending pharyngeal artery, middle meningeal artery, and artery of pterygoid canal.

Tympanic plexus (the bony part) and branch of sphenopalatine nerve (V)

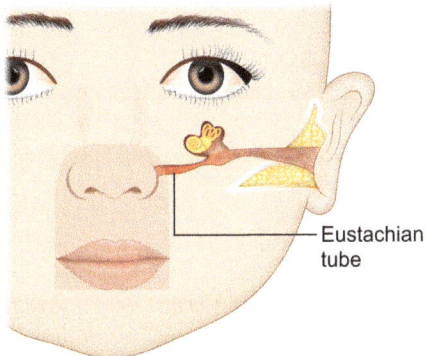

Fig. 7: Infantile Eustachian tube, which has an angle of 10° with the horizontal.

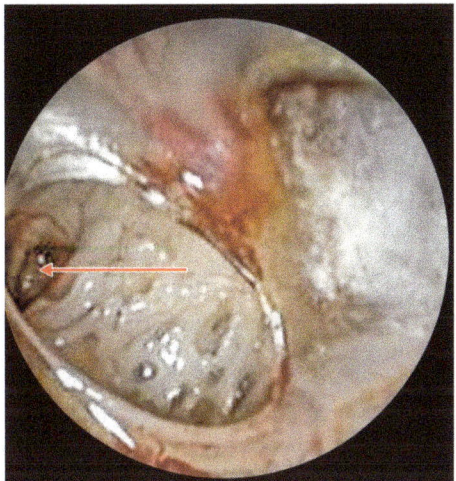

Fig. 9: Eustachian tube orifice (red arrow) seen through the central perforation.

- Patulous Eustachian tube—(patent tube). It occurs due to Ostmann's pad fat atrophy after substantial weight loss or postpregnancy. Patient has symptoms of autophonia and aural fullness.

Eustachian Tube Dysfunction

It is due to chronic inflammation, abnormal obstruction, failure of dilatation due to muscle problems **(Figs. 8 and 9)**.

- *Dilatory dynamic dysfunction:* Strong factor in Eustachian tube disorders in infants
- *Anatomical obstruction:* Adenoid hypertrophy and nasopharynx tumors
- Intrinsic blockage occurs due to allergy or laryngopharyngeal reflux.

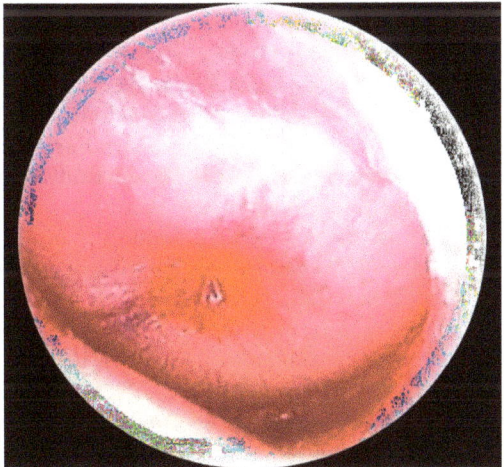

Fig. 8: Acute otitis media common in children due to Eustachian tube dysfunction.

(cartilaginous part) innervates the Eustachian tube.
- In children, the Eustachian tube is around 18 mm in length, half of the adult size **(Fig. 7)**.
- Bony part of the Eustachian tube remains patent and the cartilaginous part is normally closed and open only for a brief period of time. So, this blocks the nasopharyngeal secretion or gastric secretion from entering the middle ear.
- Short period of interval of the opening of the Eustachian tube provides ventilation.

■ BIBLIOGRAPHY

1. Bylander A, Tjernstrom O, Ivarsson A. Pressure opening and closing functions of the Eustachian tube by inflation and deflation in children and adults with normal ears. Acta Otolaryngol (Stockh). 1983;96:255-68.
2. Bylander A, Tjernstrom O. Changes in Eustachian tube function with age in children

with normal ears: a longitudinal study. Acta Otolaryngol (Stockh). 1983;96:467-77.
3. Graves GO, Edwards LF. The Eustachian tube: review of its descriptive, microscopic, topographic, and clinical anatomy. Arch Otolaryngol. 1944;39:359-97.
4. Ishijima K, Sando I, Balaban C, Suzuki C, Takasaki K. Length of the Eustachian tube and its postnatal development: computer-aided three dimensional reconstruction and measurement study. Ann Otol Rhinol Laryngol. 2000;109:542-8.
5. Ishijima K, Sando I, Miura M, Balaban CD, Takasaki K, Sudo M. Postnatal development of static volume of the Eustachian tube lumen. Ann Otol Rhinol Laryngol. 2002;111:832-5.
6. Lim DJ. Functional morphology of the tubotympanum. Acta Otolaryngol (Stockh). 1984;98 (Suppl 414):13-8.
7. Matsune S, Sando I, Takahashi H. Comparative study of elastic at the hinge portion of Eustachian tube cartilage in normal and cleft palate individuals. In: Lim DJ, Bluestone CD, Klein JO, et al. (Eds). Recent Advances in Otitis Media: Proceedings of the Fifth International Symposium. Burlington: BC Decker; 1993. pp. 4-6.
8. Mondain M, Vidal D, Bouhanna S, Uziel A. Monitoring Eustachian tube opening: Preliminary results in normal subjects. Laryngoscope. 1997;107:1414-9.
9. Orita Y, Sando I, Hasebe S, Miura M. Postnatal change on the location of Ostmann's fatty tissue in the region lateral to Eustachian tube. Int J Pediatr Otorhinolaryngol. 2003;67:1105-12.
10. Prades JM, Dumollard JM, Calloc'h F, Merzougui N, Veyret C, Martin C. Descriptive anatomy of the human auditory tube. Surg Radiol Anat. 1998;20(5):335-40.
11. Proctor B. Embryology and anatomy of the Eustachian tube. Arch Otolaryngol. 1967;86:503-26.
12. Sadler-Kimes D, Siegel MI, Todhunter JS. Age-related morphologic differences in the components of the Eustachian tube/middle-ear system. Ann Otol Rhinol Laryngol. 1989;98:854-8.
13. Sando I, Takahashi H, Matsune S, Aoki H. Localization of function in the Eustachian tube: a hypothesis. Ann Otol Rhinol Laryngol. 1993;103:311-4.
14. Siegel MI, Cantekin EI, Todhunter JS, Sadler-Kimes D. Aspect ratio as a descriptor of Eustachian tube cartilage shape. Ann Otol Rhinol Laryngol. 1988;97 (Suppl 133):16-7.
15. Siegel MI, Sadler-Kimes D, Todhunter JS. ET cartilage shape as a factor in the epidemiology of otitis media. In: Lim DJ, Bluestone CD, Klein JO, Nelson JD (Eds). Recent Advances in Otitis Media: Proceedings of the Fourth International Symposium. Burlington: BC Decker; 1988. pp. 114-7.
16. Sudo M, Sando I, Ikui A, Suzuki C. Narrowest (isthmus) portion of Eustachian tube: a computer-aided three-dimensional reconstruction and measurement study. Ann Otol Rhinol Laryngol. 1997;106:583-8.
17. Suzuki C, Balaban CD, Sando I, Sudo M, Ganbo T, Kitagawa M. Postnatal development of Eustachian tube: a computer-aided 3-D reconstruction and measurement study. Acta Otolaryngol (Stockh). 1998;118:837-43.
18. Swarts JD, Rood SR, Doyle WJ. Fetal development of the auditory tube and paratubal musculature. Cleft Palate J. 1986;23:289-311.
19. Tos M, Bak-Pedersen K. Goblet cell population in the normal middle ear and Eustachian tube of children and adults. Ann Otol Rhinol Laryngol. 1976;85 (Suppl 25):44-50.
20. Tos M. Growth of the fetal Eustachian tube and its dimensions. Arch Klin Exp Ohren Nasen Kehlkopfheilkd. 1971;198:177-86.
21. Wolff D. The microscopic anatomy of the Eustachian tube. Ann Otol Rhinol Laryngol. 1934;43:483.

CHAPTER 6

Radiology of the Temporal Bone

■ INTRODUCTION (FIGS. 1A TO D)

Magnetic resonance imaging (MRI) and computed tomography (CT) scan are the most used imaging modalities to study the temporal bone, central auditory pathways, and vestibular pathways. Therefore, it is important for otology surgeons to know about the advantages, drawbacks, and clinical correlation of MRI and CT scan. It is necessary as it will enable surgeons to choose appropriate modalities considering the nature and the status of the pathology.

Computed tomography scan is superior to MRI in terms of spatial resolution and the contrast it provides between bone, soft tissue, and air. Multislice high-resolution CT allows precise demonstration of delicate middle ear structures such as ossicles, facial nerve, spaces of retrotympanum, and the inner ear. Preoperative identification, such as the extension of disease, erosion of ossicular chain, labyrinthine fistula, exposed dura, exposed facial nerve, and ossification, helps plan the surgery (management) and helps reduce

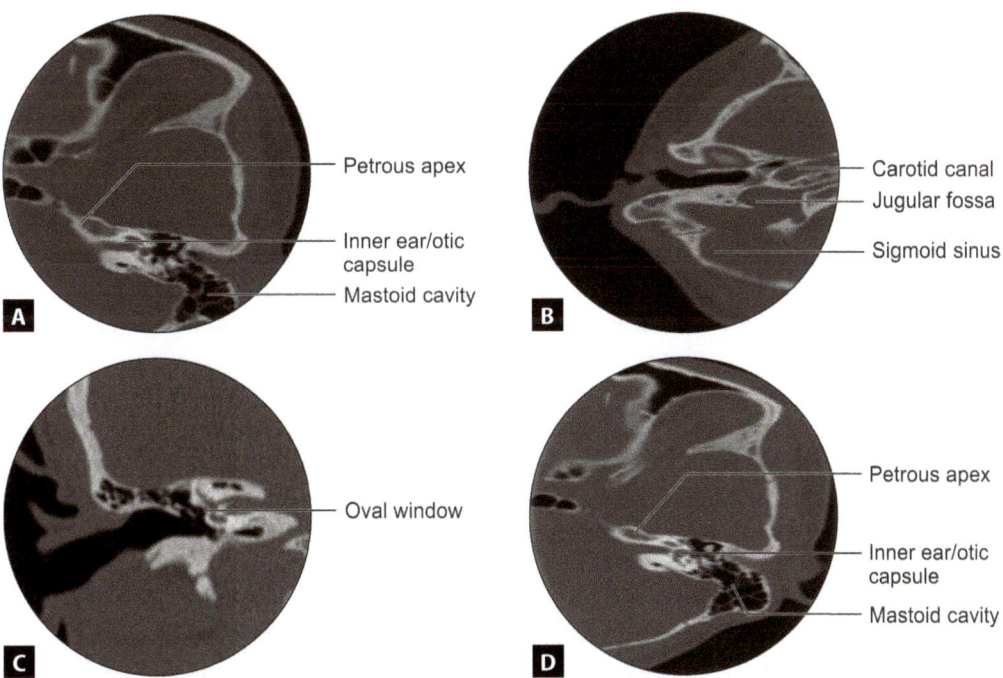

Figs. 1A to D: Radiology of the temporal bone.

TABLE 1: Interpretations of commonly used magnetic resonance imagings (MRIs).

Content	T1	T2	T1 gadolinium-enhanced
Fat	Hyperintense	Hyperintense	Hyperintense
Watery mucus	Hypointense	Hyperintense	Hypointense
Protein-rich mucus	Hyperintense	Hyperintense	Hyperintense
Concentrated mucus	Hypointense	Hypointense	Hypointense
Tumor	Medium (as muscle)	Hyperintense	Hyperintense
Air and bone	No signal	No signal	No signal/hypointense

the surgical risks. CT also identifies variations such as low middle fossa, low dura, high jugular bulb, and pneumatization. Lack of signal from the bone and insufficient spatial resolution in MRI limit it to identify the middle ear structures.

Magnetic resonance imaging, on the other hand, is supreme in the contrast between soft tissues which is necessary for making the differential diagnosis and identifying the staging of the neoplasm. MRI is also advantageous over the CT scan to see recurrence or residual disease in the middle ear cleft after the removal of cholesteatoma. In CT scans, it is not always possible to discriminate between residual cholesteatoma and postoperative surgical changes.

Table 1 shows the interpretation of T1, T2, and T1 gadolinium-enhanced MRIs.

The two submodalities used in MRI are:
1. *Fat suppression:* It is commonly used in MRI to suppress the signal coming from adipose tissue or detect adipose tissue. It is recommended to stop large amounts of fat cells from acquiring reliable contrast material-enhanced images.
   a. *Advantages:*
      i. Lipid-specific is better for contrast-enhancing T1 images, especially in areas with significant fat.
      ii. Avoids artifacts due to chemical shifts.
      iii. Allows good visualization of small anatomic details.
   b. *Disadvantages:*
      i. It relies on the frequency of the pulse, which should equate to the frequency of lipid. Inhomogeneity causes inadequate fat suppression and sometimes water suppression.
      ii. Naturally occurring water in adipose tissue is not saturated. Fraction of fatty acid with resonance as water remains unsuppressed.
2. *Diffusion-weighted imaging:* It is a contrast imaging sequence. The contrast occurs from the differences in the motion of water molecules and tissues.
   a. *Advantages:*
      i. Quick to perform.
      ii. Gives knowledge about tumor detection and characterization.
      iii. It helps see the tumors' response to treatment and predicts the course of treatment.
   b. *Disadvantages:*
      i. More research is needed.
      ii. Requires standardization of data acquisitions and analysis.

CLINICAL ASPECTS
- CT scan details bony structures better while MRI is superior to CT for soft tissue visualizations.
- Both CT and MRI are essential to evaluate the extratemporal extension of a pathological condition.

For CT scan all the three cuts: Axial, coronal, and sagittal are important.
- *Both axial and sagittal cuts show better:* The pneumatization of mastoid and the dural and sigmoid level.
- The entire course of the facial nerve is better appreciated in coronal and axial cuts.
- Both axial and coronal cuts are required to judge the extent of cholesteatoma (medial/lateral to ossicles) and hence aids in preoperative planning.
- *Coronal cuts become inevitable for pathologies like:* Epitympanum cholesteatoma, involvement of Prussack's space, scutum erosion and lateral semicircular canal (LSC) fistula.
- *Axial cuts are most sought after for findings like:* Dehiscence of wall between carotid canal and cochlea, erosion of keel area in glomus jugulare and for better assessment of jugular foramen, sinus tympani, and facial recess.

■ AXIAL SECTIONS

To avoid missing pathological findings, it is essential to observe the entire temporal bone.
- The top of the superior semicircular canal (SCC; elliptical) is visualized as a line of two dots anterolateral and posteromedially with the upper part of the mastoid process **(Fig. 2)**.
- The subarcuate artery arises from the posterior cranial fossa and passes through the superior SCC (same as the subarcuate cell tract) **(Fig. 3)**.
- Superior end of the posterior SCC and posterior end of the superior SCC seen as crus commune **(Fig. 4)**.
- Superior aspect of the internal auditory meatus (IAM) with cochlea and vestibule

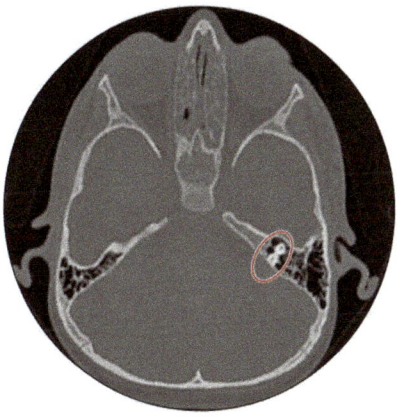
Fig. 2: The superior semicircular canal (SCC).

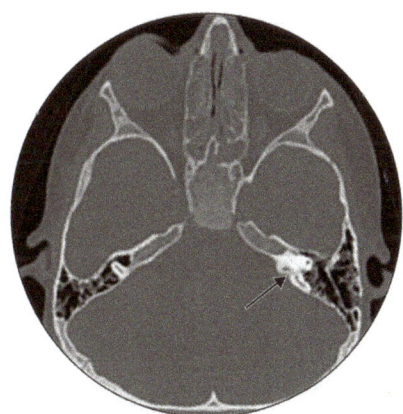
Fig. 3: The subarcuate artery.

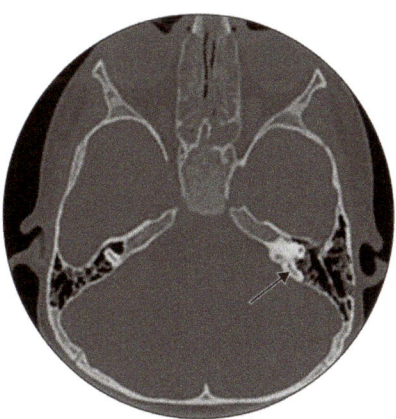
Fig. 4: The crus commune.

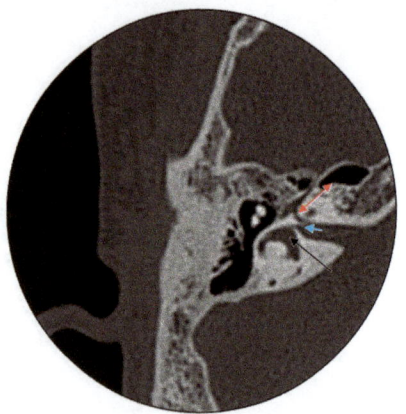

Fig. 5: The cochlea with the upper part of internal auditory meatus (IAM).

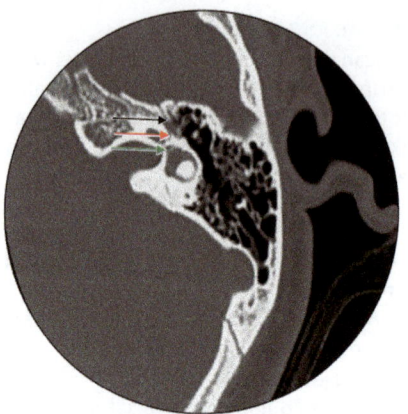

Fig. 7: The facial nerve and superior vestibular nerve.

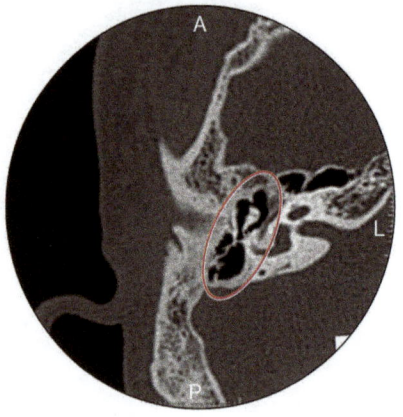

Fig. 6: Mastoid antrum, aditus, and attic region.

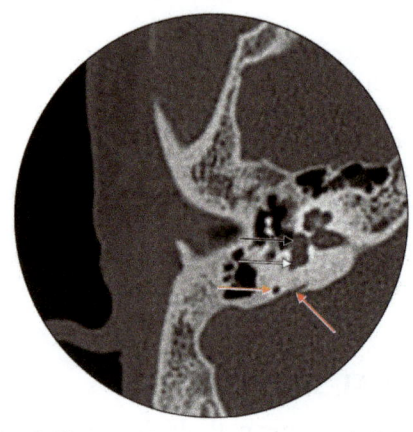

Fig. 8: The superior semicircular canals (SCCs).

[superior part (arrow)] seen with the labyrinthine facial nerve (arrowhead). The vertical crest of the IAM is visualized clearly (red double arrow) **(Fig. 5)**.
- Hourglass appearance of the attic, aditus, and antrum and the superior aspect of the ossicle (elliptical marking) are visualized (anteriorly head of the malleus, posteriorly body incus) **(Fig. 6)**.
- Geniculate ganglion (black arrow) visualized anteromedial to the ossicles. Division within the lateral part of IAM visualized clearly [facial nerve (red arrow)], superior vestibular nerve (green arrow) **(Fig. 7)**.
- Ampulla of lateral SCC (white arrow) and the ampulla of superior SCC entry into the vestibule (black arrow) with lateral SCC are visualized. Posterior to posterior SCC (orange arrow), the channel of the vestibular aqueduct (red arrow) is seen clearly **(Fig. 8)**.
- Posterior epitympanum with cone and ice cream shape of ossicles (elliptical marking) with horizontal facial nerve (black arrow) anteromedially with lateral

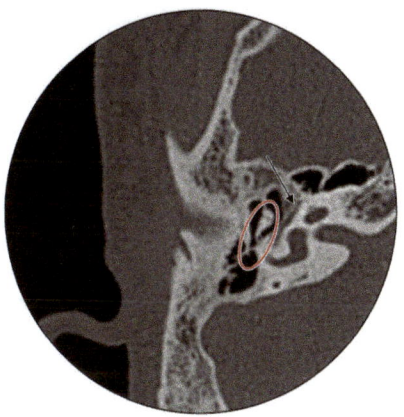

Fig. 9: The ossicles and the tympanic part of the facial nerve.

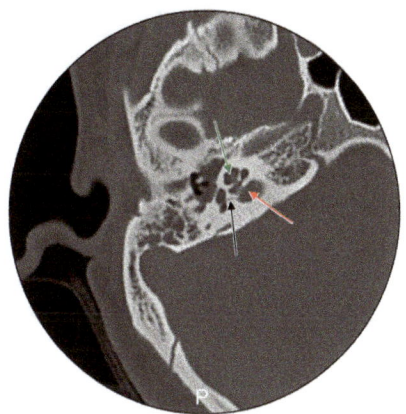

Fig. 10: The cochlea, vestibule, and singular nerve.

SCC and short process of incus relations can be seen. Pneumatization of mastoid cells with supracochlear air cells can be seen in this view **(Fig. 9)**.
- Level of the horizontal facial nerve with cochleariform process and scala of the cochlea (green arrow) with vestibule and lower aspect of IAM are visualized (red arrow). Ampulla of posterior SCC and vestibule with vestibular aqueduct are seen. Singular nerve (black arrow) can be visualized in the lower part of IAM (red arrow) **(Fig. 10)**.

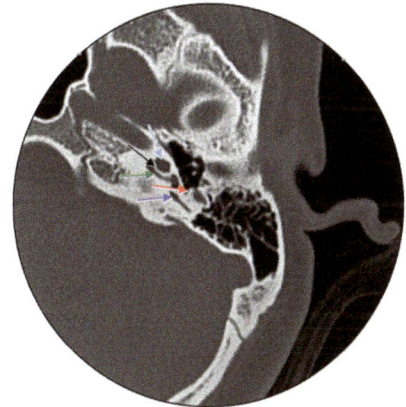

Fig. 11: The pyramidal eminence.

CLINICAL ASPECT
Cuts involving the lowest part of basal turn of cochlea should be visualized, in cases of ossificans before cochlear implantation, as this is the site to get involved first.

- Pyramidal eminence (red arrow) from which the tendon of stapedius muscle emerges from the anterior face of the vertical facial nerve. The ampullary end of the posterior SCC (purple arrow) is located near the bottom of the tympanic sinus. The axis of the cochlea is directed anterolaterally, and the basal turn of the cochlea (green arrow) is divided from the apical two turns (blue arrow) by thick bone (black arrow) **(Fig. 11)**.
- *Round window niche (red arrow):* The border between the inner ear fluid in the basal turn and the air in the place corresponds to the round window membrane. The lateral soft tissue bundle in the posterior wall of the tympanic cavity corresponds to the facial nerve (green arrow), and the medial one is the stapedius muscle (orange arrow) **(Fig. 12)**.

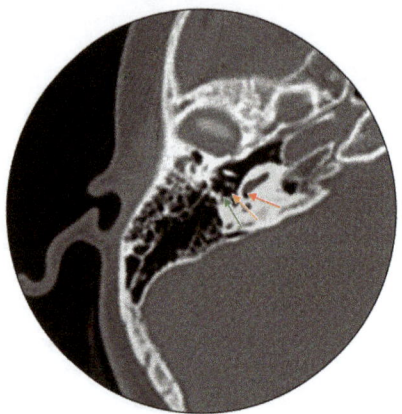 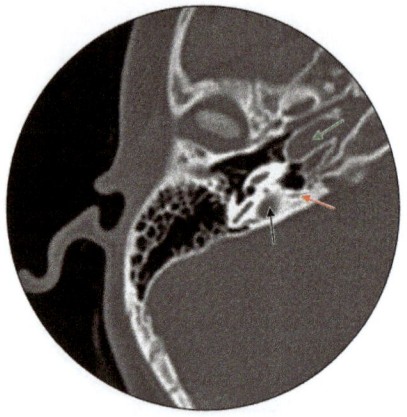

Fig. 12: The round window niche.

Fig. 13: The jugular bulb and carotid artery.

CLINICAL ASPECT
Round window area is visualized:
- To look for obliteration and ossification at that level.
- To assess the position of round window for cochlear implantation and look for chorda tympani and facial nerve angle.
- To look for any dehiscence of jugular bulb and plan for extended facial recess approach if required.

- Jugular bulb starts to visualize, cochlear aqueduct (red arrow) is pictured between the cochlea and jugular bulb. It connects the scala tympani to the subarachnoid space. In the hypotympanum, we can see the carotid canal anteromedially (green arrow), the jugular bulb posterolaterally (black arrow), and thick bone of cochlea is caught in between. We can also visualize infracochlear pathways to petrous apex in many CT scans **(Fig. 13)**.

■ CORONAL SECTIONS

- The level of vertical segment of the internal carotid artery and protympanum can be visualized **(Fig. 14)**.
- Cochlear turn (purple arrow), scutum (red arrow), ossicles (blue arrow), geniculate ganglion, and horizontal facial nerve

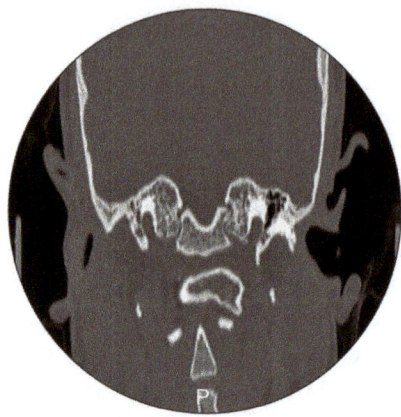

Fig. 14: Coronal computed tomography (CT) scan with protympanum area.

(green arrow) along with tegmen tympani and supracochlear air cells are visualized in the slice **(Fig. 15)**.
- The bony shell located at the bottom of the bony depression between facial nerve and promontory corresponds to the oval window. The footplate forms the lateral wall of the vestibule (green arrow), while the medial wall forms the lateral wall of the IAM (red arrow) **(Fig. 16)**.
- Ampulla of superior and lateral SCC are visualized with the air-fluid demarcation in the round window niche. The horizontal crest (arrow) divides the IAM **(Fig. 17)**.

Radiology of the Temporal Bone

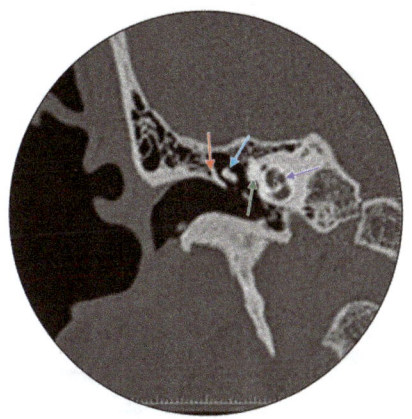

Fig. 15: Areas from scutum to cochlear turns.

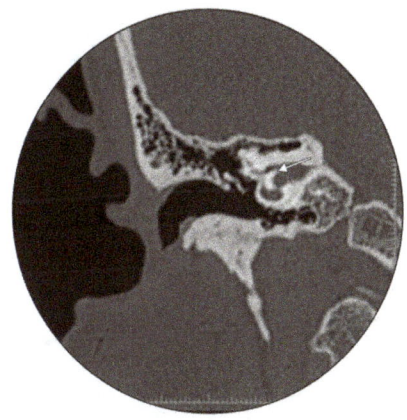

Fig. 17: The internal auditory meatus (IAM) with its horizontal crest.

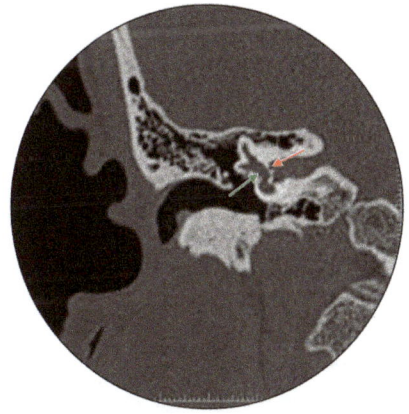

Fig. 16: The vestibule and internal auditory meatus (IAM).

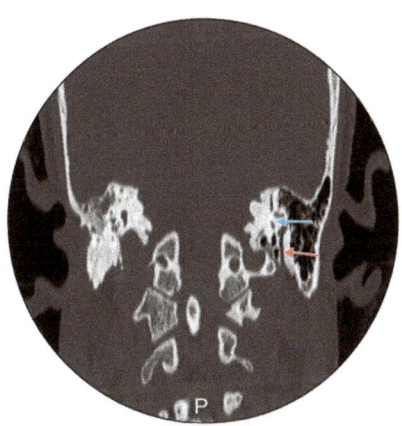

Fig. 18: The mastoid segment of the facial nerve.

- The facial nerve (red arrow) coarses inferomedially to the lateral SCC (blue arrow). The stapedius muscle turns medially to the facial nerve, and the tympanic sinus is located medially to the pyramidal eminence and muscle. The ampulla of the posterior SCC is located at the bottom of the tympanic sinus **(Fig. 18)**.

To visualize any structure in detail on a high-resolution computed tomography (HRCT) temporal bone, it is advisable to do a three-dimensional (3D) reconstruction by keeping in view all the sections of the CT scan.

Below are the images of the oblique sagittal section of the HRCT temporal bone.
- Facial nerve and the lateral SCC **(Fig. 19)**.
- Cochlear turns **(Fig. 20)**.
- Jugular bulb as seen on oblique sagittal **(Fig. 21)**.

DEVELOPMENTAL VARIATIONS

Anatomical variations in size and position of several components of the temporal bone are common.
- *Mastoid:* Development of the mastoid varies from person to person and from side to side in the same individual.

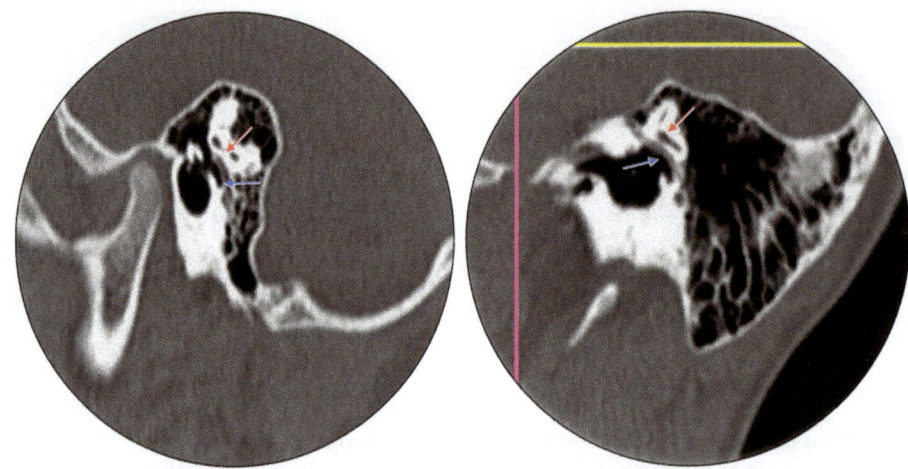

Fig. 19: The facial nerve (blue arrow) and lateral SCC (red arrow).

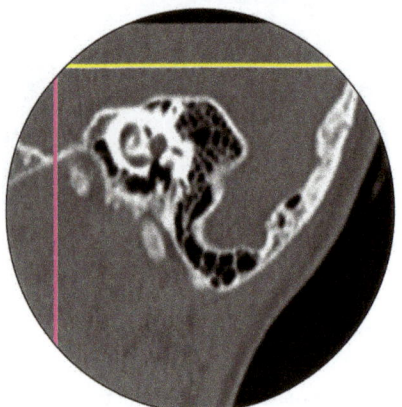

Fig. 20: The cochlear turns (arrow).

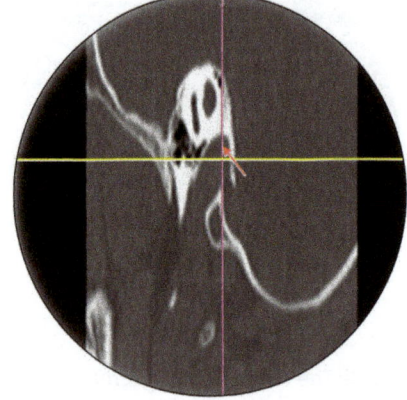

Fig. 21: The jugular bulb (red arrow).

- *Lateral sinus (sigmoid):* Anterior location of sigmoid sinus appears in many mastoids.
- *Tegmen:* The tegmen of the mastoid and attic are usually oriented in the horizontal plane, slightly lower than arcuate eminence. Variation in the dural plate (lower or depressed) is seen in congenital atresia.
- *Jugular fossa:* There is tremendous variation in the size of the jugular fossa and the jugular bulb. Deviations may be present from patient to patient and from side to side of the same individual. For the translabyrinthine approach and retrofacial approach, one should know the level of the jugular bulb. A dehiscent jugular bulb is also frequently seen.
- *Carotid artery:* Minor variations are seen in the intratemporal course of ICA. It might take an ectopic route from the middle ear. This anomaly should be recognized before surgery. Anomalous ICA may enter through an enlarged inferior canaliculus or via an opening in the floor of the posterior aspect of the hypotympanum.

- *Arachnoid granulation:* This villous structure herniates through minor defects in the dura and drains cerebrospinal fluid (CSF) from subarachnoid space into the venous system. A variable number of arachnoid granulations do not reach their venous target but come in contact with the intracranial surface of the middle ear cleft. Over time the pulsation of the CSF may produce small areas of bone resorption and erosion. It is clinically significant when they open into the adjacent air spaces (attic, mastoid air cells) and produce CSF otorrhea.
- *Petrous apex:* It may be pneumatized, diploic, or compact.

A good CT study provides the surgeon with essential information about the feasibility of corrective surgery.
- Degree and type of tympanic bone abnormality
- Pneumatization of the mastoid and air cells
- The development and the aeration of the middle ear cavity
- The status of the ossicular chain
- The patency of the labyrinthine windows
- The facial nerve canal
- The development of inner ear structures (modiolus and spiral lamina)
- Intracranial relations and variations.

It is essential to know the limitation of radiological diagnosis. Blind confidence in the radiological report is entirely inappropriate. To avoid misdiagnosis, the surgeon should be prepared himself to interpret the radiogram. These two modalities, CT scan, and MRI are currently complimentary to each other, and the surgeon needs to choose the right one or both, for proper management.

CLINICAL ASPECT
- For cochlear implantation, it is important to look for modiolar view to: (1) View cochlear aperture and cochlear nerve. (2) Look for presence of modiolus. (3) To study the morphology of all the cochlear turns.
- *For any cochlear implantation:* CT is required, but the most inevitable radiology is MRI of temporal bone and inner ear.

Below is a depiction of various typical structures of temporal bone seen on HRCT temporal bone **(Fig. 22)**.

PATHOLOGICAL CONDITIONS

Pathological conditions such as congenital malformations, trauma, inflammation, neoplasms, and otodystrophies show peculiar changes in the temporal bone radiological investigations. An MRI temporal bone is often required to assess the pathological conditions which spread outside the vicinity of the pneumatized temporal bone.

Congenital Malformations
- *Congenital anomalies of the temporal bone:* A proper imaging assessment is essential in congenital anomalies, precisely in the anomalies of the sound conducting system and inner ear anomalies. A good CT scan will provide the surgeon with the following basic information:
  - The degree and the type of abnormality of the temporal bone (minor deformity to complete agenesis)
  - Pneumatization of the middle ear cleft
  - Development of the middle ear cavity including aeration and ossicular status (size, shape, persistence, or fusion)
  - The course of the facial nerve
  - The labyrinthine windows
  - Development of the inner ear structures
  - Status of the tegmen and the sinuses.

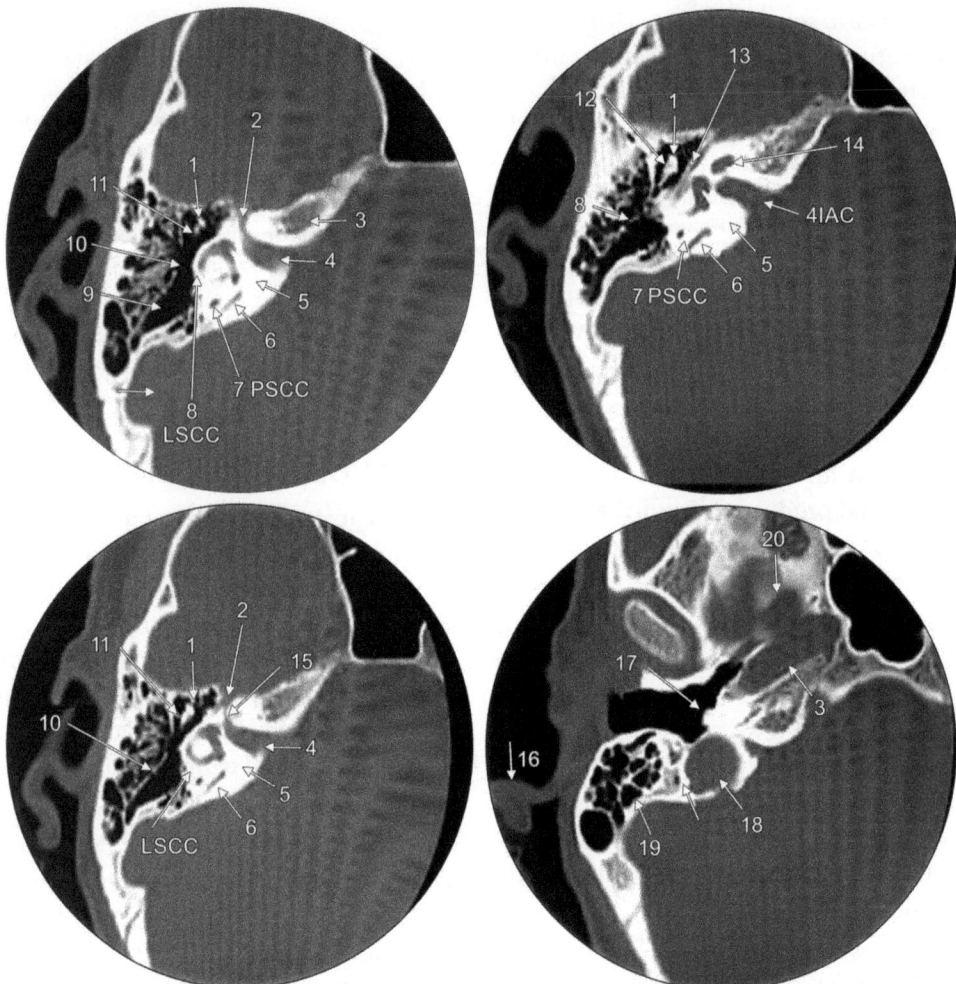

Fig. 22: Various typical anatomical structures are seen on high-resolution computed tomography (HRCT) temporal bone. (1: Head of malleus; 2: Geniculate ganglion; 3: Internal carotid artery; 4: Internal auditory canal; 5: Otic capsule; 6: Vestibular aqueduct; 7: PSCC; 8: LSCC; 9: Mastoid antrum; 10: Korner's septum; 11: Body of incus; 12: Incudomalleal joint; 13: Tympanic part of facial nerve; 14: Apical turn of cochlea; 15: Labyrinthine segment of facial nerve; 16: Pinna; 17: Lower part of basal turn of cochlea; 18: Jugular bulb; 19: Sigmoid sinus; 20: Eustachian tube).

- *Anomalies of the ear for the sensorineural deafness:* Bony otic capsule is visualized in the CT scan, while membranous labyrinth requires MRI.
  - Anomalies of the cochlear duct, the vestibule, and the semicircular canal with vestibular and cochlear aqueduct
  - Assessment of the IAM with all four nerve segments
- *Anomalies of the facial nerve:* It shows complete or partial agenesis of the facial nerve with total paralysis, sometimes narrow and hypoplastic facial nerve. The horizontal segment is displaced inferiorly

to cover the oval window. Anomalies of the vertical component are common in congenital external ear atresia.

Temporal Bone Trauma

It usually occurs with a head injury. So, one must rule out CSF rhinorrhea, CSF otorrhea, facial nerve paralysis/profound deafness, and vertigo. Fractures are of two types according to the extent of involvement along the axis.
1. Longitudinal fracture transverse fracture **(Fig. 23)**
2. Longitudinal fractures are best demonstrated in the axial and sagittal scans.

Transverse fractures are best seen in the axial and sagittal scans (transverse fracture crosses the petrous pyramid perpendicular to the long axis of the pyramid). Traumatic disruption of the ossicles is seen in the longitudinal fractures. The presence of air in the vestibule indicates rupture of the stapes.
- Labyrinthine concussion and bleeding
  Magnetic resonance imaging is required for injured membranous part of the labyrinth, leading to irreversible deafness and transient vestibular symptoms.

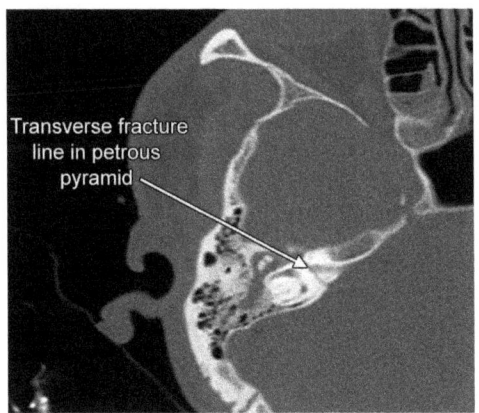

Fig. 23: Transverse fracture line (It involves temporal squama, mastoid, epitympanum).

- Traumatic facial palsy
  Complete transaction of the facial nerve. Delayed facial palsy occurs due to post-traumatic edema. With a CT scan evaluation of the course of the fracture line, the site of the lesion can be determined.
- Meningocele and meningoencephalocele
  It is due to injury to the tegmen, which leads to fracture, and the defect leads to meningoencephalocele. In MRI, a meningocele has a signal identical to the CSF. The appearance of encephalocele is similar to that of the brain.

Inflammatory Conditions

- *Acute otomastoiditis:* This presents as a homogenous opacification of the middle ear and the mastoid, subperiosteal abscess, and erosion of the tegmen and the sinus may develop.
- *Chronic otomastoiditis:* CSOM shows typical radiological findings **(Fig. 24)**
  - Thickening of the mastoid trabeculae
  - Inhomogeneous opacification of the air cells
  - Erosion of the ossicles.
- *Malignant necrotizing otitis:* Pseudomonas bacteria cause osteomyelitis of the temporal bone. CT scan is excellent for demonstrating the involvement of the external ear, the middle ear, the petrous pyramid, and MRI is necessary for the facial nerve involvement or involvement beyond the confines of the temporal bone.
- *Labyrinthitis:* In contrast to MRI, enhancement is seen within the lumen of the bony labyrinth (viral/bacterial labyrinthitis) due to damage of the capillary endothelium, which leads to a disruption of the labyrinth-blood barrier. Chronic labyrinthitis suggests local/focal erosion of the lumen of the inner

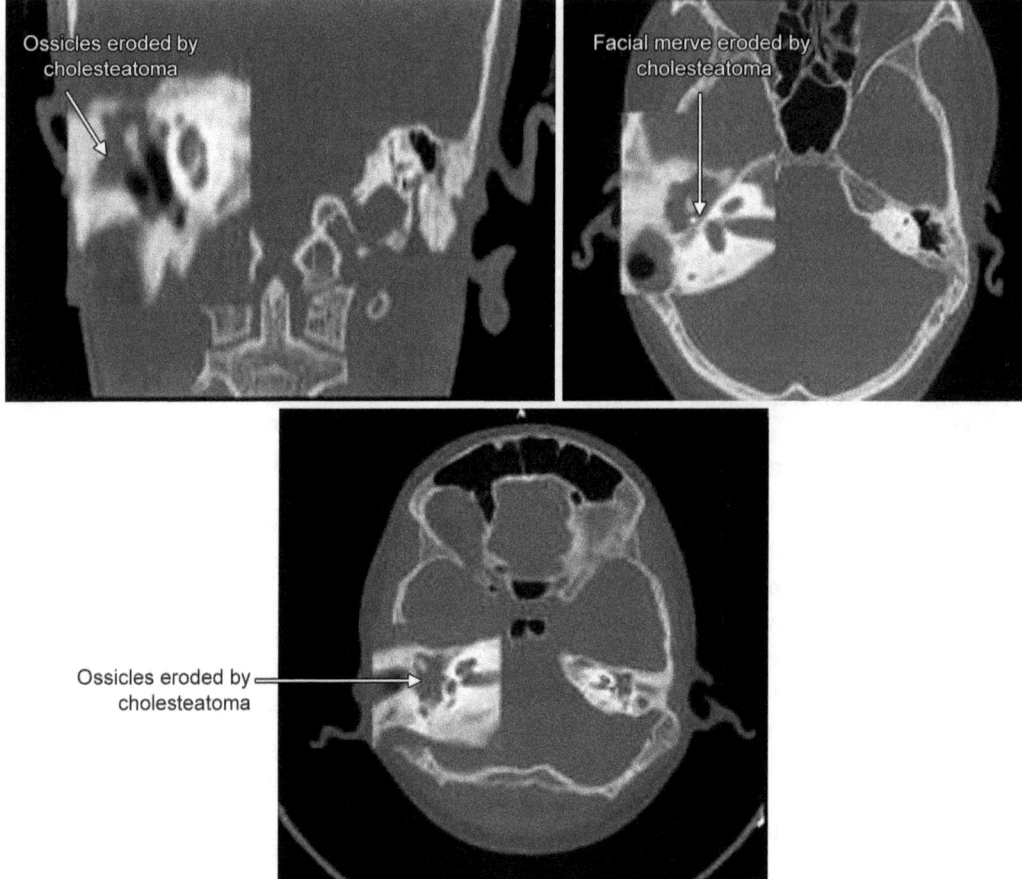

Fig. 24: Computed tomography (CT) scan showing the effects of chronic otomastoiditis.

ear, which is filled with (partially/totally) granulation and leads to fibrosis and obliteration of the lumen.
- *Neuritis:* Unilateral or bilateral involvement is seen in anterior genu (in the Bell's palsy or Ramsay-Hunt syndrome) on MRI, with varying degrees of enhancement.
- *Cholesteatoma:* Erosion of the ossicles, the dura, the sinus, the facial nerve, and structures of the inner ear. The inner ear is seen with a CT scan. The fistula in the ampullary end of the lateral semicircular canal is seen as flattening the medial wall of the posterior epitympanum. Displacement of the ossicles (medial/lateral), soft tissue opacity seen in spaces of the retrotympanum, and extension of disease in the pneumatic portion of the temporal bone (supracochlear, infracochlear, perilabyrinthine, retrofacial, Trautmann's triangle, etc.).

Congenital Cholesteatoma

Computed tomography examination shows a well-defined soft tissue mass within the middle ear, opacification of the tympanic cavity, bulging of the tympanic membrane, and erosion of the ossicles. MRI may help identify the presence and size of the cholesteatoma.

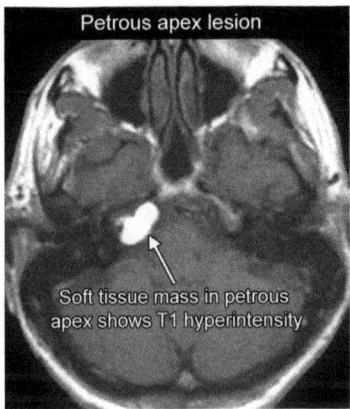

Fig. 25: Cholesteatoma of petrous apex.

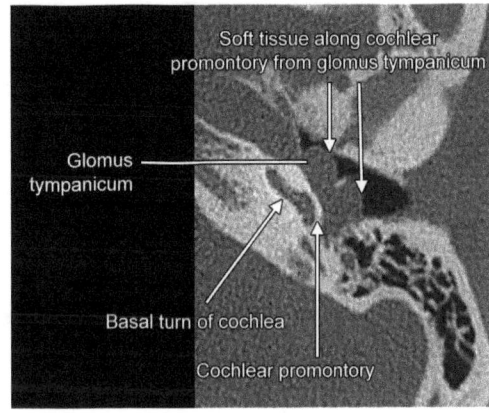

Fig. 26: Computed tomography (CT) scan showing glomus tympanicum.

Petrous Apex Cholesteatoma

Computed tomography scan shows **(Fig. 25)**:
- Expansile cystic lesion
- Expansion of the involved pyramid
- Elevated and thinned superior petrous ridge
- As the lesion expands, the IAM and the labyrinth are eroded.
- Cholesteatoma arising from the epidural or meningeal spaces of the superior aspect of the pyramid creates a scooped-out defect of the adjacent elements of the pyramid. There is no bony rim as the lesion arises from within the pyramid.

Keratosis Obturans and Cholesteatoma of External Auditory Canal

- Enlargement of the entire circumference of the canal
- Scooped-out defect of the bony canal
- Soft tissue mass containing small bony sequestra may fill the lumen of the canal.

Neoplastic Conditions

There are two groups of neoplasms:
1. Carcinoma involving the external auditory canal, the middle ear cleft, the jugular bulb, and the petrous apex.

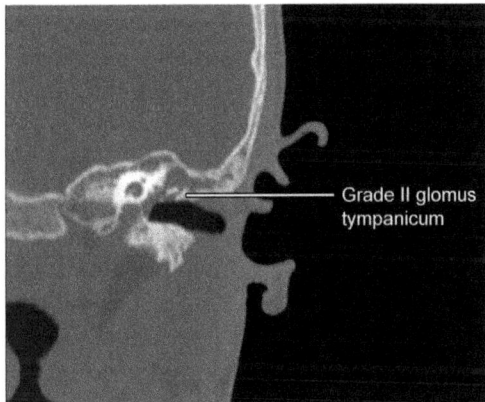

Fig. 27: Computed tomography (CT) scan showing grade II glomus tympanicum.

The carcinoma extends to and destroys structures such as mastoid, middle ear cavity, facial canal, Eustachian tube, jugular bulb, and petrous apex, giving a typical mottled or moth-eaten appearance of the bone.

2. Neuroma, glomus tumors, and meningioma
    a. *Glomus tumors:*
        i. *Glomus tympanicum (Figs. 26 and 27):* In axial/coronal CT scan, it is seen as a well-defined and enhancing soft tissue mass in the lower part of the tympanic cavity.

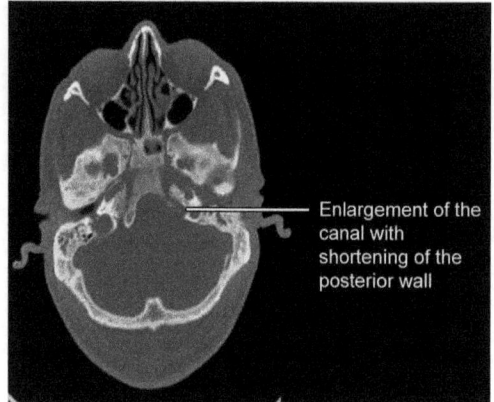

Fig. 28: Computed tomography (CT) scan showing vestibular schwannoma.

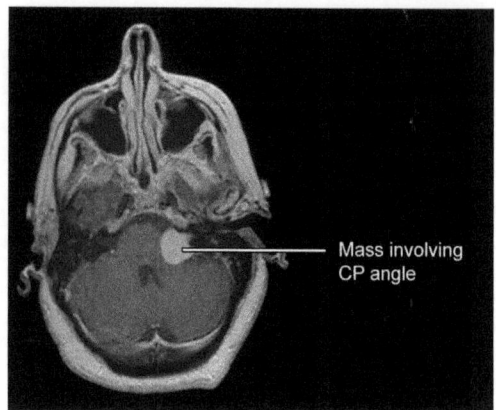

Fig. 29: Magnetic resonance imaging (MRI) showing cerebellopontine (CP) angle mass.

It may extend to the mastoid, the hypotympanum, and the carotid.
  b. *Glomus jugulare:* MRI is the investigation of choice.
     i. Enlarged jugular bulb with the erosion of the cortical bone and bony septum separating the jugular bulb and the internal carotid artery.
     ii. Asymmetry of the jugular bulb.
     iii. Extension to the middle ear cleft and the external auditory meatus.
     iv. Erosion of the facial nerve.
     v. Inner ear extension with the petrous bone involvement.
     vi. Extracranial involvement.
  c. *Vestibular schwannoma* **(Figs. 28 and 29):** Gadolinium-enhanced MRI is the choice of the investigation.
     i. Complete study of the IAM (T1, T2)
     ii. Fat suppression images are required for recurrence or history of removal of the tumors that have fat-containing graft.
     iii. CT scan
     iv. Comparison of the two IAMs
     v. Enlargement of the canal with shortening of the posterior wall **(Fig. 28)**.
  d. Meningiomas
     Magnetic resonance imaging: En plaque lesions appear as focal areas of enhancing, thick meninges. The meningeal involvement often extends from the actual tumor mass, producing tail signs.

Otodystrophies

- *Otosclerosis:*
  - Axial and 20° coronal oblique sections (1 mm thickness)
  - Loss of definition of the margin of the oval window to narrowing and obliteration of the oval window
  - Postoperative dislodgement of the prosthesis into the vestibule
  - Separation of the implant from the incus
  - Reobliteration of the oval window with fixation of the strut.
- *Cochlear otosclerosis (Fig. 30):*
  - Progressive enlargement of the perifenestral pocket or as a single or multiple foci in the other locations of the cochlea and the labyrinthine capsule.
  - The regular cochlear capsule is disrupted in the cochlear otosclerosis.

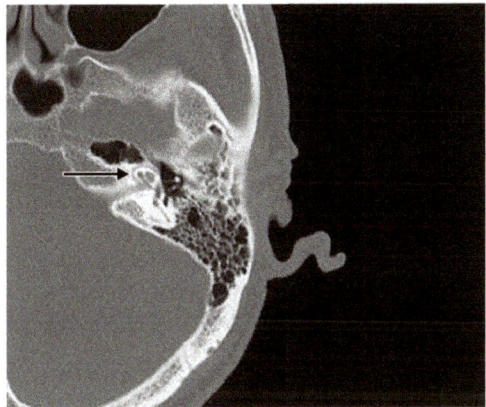

Fig. 30: Cochlear otosclerosis (arrow).

- A typical sign is the formation of a band of demineralization surrounding the cochlear canal (double ring effect).
- Active stage shows hypervascularity as a hyperintense lesion and lacunae found in the foci.

CLINICAL ASPECT
- Otosclerosis though is a clinical diagnosis, imaging helps in supporting the diagnosis, presurgical planning, and to assess the recurrence of symptoms.
- The CT findings in otosclerosis depend on the stage of the disease and the area involved by the disease.

BIBLIOGRAPHY

1. Antonelli Pl, Garside JA, Mancusso AA, Strickler ST, Kubilis PS. Computed tomography and the diagnosis of coalescent mastoiditis. Otolaryngol Head Neck Surg. 1999;120(3):350-4.
2. Bamiou DE. Phelps P, Sirimanna T. Temporal bone computed tomography findings in bilateral sensorineural hearing loss. Arch Dis Child. 2000;82(3):257-60.
3. Boston M, Halstead M. Meinzen-Derr J, Bean J, Vijayasekaran S, Arjmand E, et al. The large vestibular aqueduct: a new definition based on audiologic and computed tomography correlation. Otolaryngol Head Neck Surg. 2007;136(6):972-7.
4. Buckingham RA, Valvassori GE. Inner ear fluid volumes and the resolution power of MRI. Ann Otol Rhinol Laryngol. 2001;110(2):113-7.
5. Casselman JW, Kulweide R, Deimling M, Ampe W, Dehaene I, Meeus L. Constructive interference in steady state-3DFT MR imaging of the inner ear and cerebellopontine angle. AJNR Am J Neuroradiol. 1993;14(1):47-57.
6. Dubrulle F, Ernst O, Vincent C, Vaneecloo FM, Lejeune JP, Lemaitre L. Cochlear fossa enhancement at MR evaluation of vestibular schwannoma: correlation with success at hearing preservation surgery. Radiology. 2000;215(2):458-62.
7. Fitzgerald DC, Mark AS. Sudden hearing loss: frequency of abnormal findings on contrast-enhanced MRI studies. AJNR Am J Neuroradial 1990;19(8):1433-6.
8. Harnsberger HR, Dahlen RT, Shelton C, Gray SD, Parkin JL. Advanced techniques in magnetic resonance imaging in the evaluation of the large endolymphatic duct and sac syndrome. Larynguscupe, 1995;105(10);1037-42.
9. Lo WW. Imaging of cochlear and auditory brain stem implantation. AJNR Am J Neuroradiol. 1998;19(6):1147-54.
10. Mackeith S, Joy R, Robinson P. Hajioff D. Pre-operative imaging for cochlear implantation: magnetic resonance imaging, computer mtomography, or both? Cochlear Implants Int. 2012;13(3):133-6.
11. Male MF, Valvassuri GE, Becker M. Imaging of Neck. New York: Thieme Verlag; 2005.
12. Mukherji SK, Albernaz VS, Lo WW, Gaffey MJ, Megerian CA, Feghali JG, et al. Papillary endolymphatic sac tumors: CT, MR imaging and angiographic findings in 20 patients. Radiology. 1997;202(3):801-8.
13. Rodgers GK, Applegate L, De La Cruz A, Lo W. Magnetic resonance angiography: analysis of vascular lesions of the temporal bone and skull base. Am J Otol. 1993;14(1):56-62.
14. Schmalbrock P, Chakeres DW, Monroe W, Saraswat A, Miles BA, Welling DB. Assessment of internal auditory canal

tuinors: a comparison of contrast enhanced T1 weighted and steady-state T2 weighted gradient echo MR imaging. AJNR Am J Neroradiol. 1999;20(7):1207-13.
15. Seltzer S, Mark AS. Contrast enhancement of the labyrinth on MR scans in patients with sudden hearing loss and vertigo: evidence of labyrinthine disease. AJNR Am J Neuroradiol. 1991;12(1):13-6.
16. Stone JA, Castillo M, Neelon B, Mukherji SK. Evaluation of CSF leaks: high resolution CT compared with contrast-enhanced CT and radionuclide cisternography. AJNR Am J Neuroradial. 1999;20(4):706-12.
17. Valvassori GE, Buckingham RA. Tomography and Cross Sections of the Ear. Philadelphia: Georg Thienie Verlag; 1975.
18. Valvassori GE, Dobben GD. CT densitometry of the cochlear capsule in otosclerosis. AJNR Am J Neuroradiol 1985;6(5):661-7.
19. Valvassori GE. The internal auditory canal revisited. The high-definition approach. Otolaryngol Clin North Am. 1995;28(3): 431-51.

Index

Page numbers followed by *f* refer to figure and *fc* refer to flowchart

A

Adenoid hypertrophy 59
Air 62
Annular ligament 24*f*
Annulus 18*f*
Anterior epitympanic
    cholesteatoma 32
    recess 12, 31, 52*f*
Arachnoid granulation 69
Arcuate eminence 6*f*
Arnold's nerve 25
Artery
    caroticotympanic 52
    subarcuate 63, 63*f*
Auditory tube 11

B

Bell's palsy 72
Bone 62
Bony external canal, skin of 14
Branchiomotor nucleus 45

C

Cadaveric dissection 34*f*
Carotid
    artery 66*f*, 68
    canal 7*f*
Cerebellar artery, anterior
    inferior 51
Cerebellopontine 9
    angle
        mass 74*f*
        surgery 17
Cerebrospinal fluid 15, 42, 51, 69
    otorrhea 71
    rhinorrhea 71
Cholesteatoma 28, 32, 72, 73
    congenital 72
    growth, embryogenic
        route of 30
    posterior
        epitympanic 31
        mesotympanic 32
    typical spread of 31
Chordal eminence 22
Chordatympani 27*f*, 52*f*
Cisternal segment 45
Citelli's angle 38
Cochlea 65*f*
    axis of 19
Cochlear
    aqueduct 7*f*
    duct, anomalies of 70
    implantation 9, 69
    otosclerosis 74, 75*f*
    turns 67, 67*f*, 68*f*
Cochleariformis process 15*f*,
    20, 48*f*
Computed tomography 17*f*, 24*f*
    examination 72
    scan 17*f*, 20*f*, 24*f*, 32*f*, 38*f*, 39,
        57*f*, 61, 72*f*-74*f*
Coronal computed tomography
    scan 66*f*
Cranial nerves 17
Crista fenestra 19
Crus commune 63

D

Deafness 71
Deep auricular artery 25
Deep sinus 28
    tympani 28
Diffusion-weighted imaging 62
Digastric ridge 53
Dilatory dynamic dysfunction 59
Diploic mastoid 40*f*

E

Ear, development of 3*f*, 11
Endolymphatic sac 38
Epithelial cells, cord of 11
Epithelial layer 18
Epitympanic retraction 32
Epitympanum 25, 33*f*, 35, 71*f*
    posterior 64
Eustachian tube 11, 12, 21, 26, 35,
    52*f*, 56, 57, 57*f*, 58, 59
    anatomy of 56
    dimensions of 57*f*
    disorders 59
    dysfunction 59
    infantile 59*f*
    mucosal lining of 58
    muscles 58*f*
    orifice 59*f*
    patulous 59
External auditory canal 4, 11,
    14, 35
    cholesteatoma of 73
External auditory meatus 8*f*, 14
External ear
    canal stenosis 11
    development of 11
External petrosquamous fissure 5
Extratemporal segment 45

F

Facial canal 45
Facial nerve 4*f*, 15, 15*f*, 20-22, 24,
    25*f*, 44, 45, 48, 50*f*, 64,
    64*f*, 66, 67, 68*f*
    anomalies of 50, 70
    arterial supply of 51
    branches of 46*f*, 49*f*
    complete transaction of 71
    development 44
    embryology of 45*f*
    intracranial course of 47*f*
    mastoid segment of 67*f*
    nuclei of 46*fc*
    paralysis 44, 71
    radiology of 44*f*

relations of 20*f*
surgical landmarks of 53, 53*f*
trajectory of 45
tympanic segment of 48, 49*f*
tympanomastoid segment of 48*f*
vasculature of 52*f*
Facial palsy, traumatic 71
Facial recess 27, 27*f*, 52, 52*f*, 63
  approach 21
  cadaveric view of 52*f*
Facial sinus 27
Fat 62
  Ostmann's pad of 57, 57*f*
  suppression 62
Fissure 9
Fistula 63
Foot plate 24*f*

G

Geniculate ganglion 15, 45, 48*f*, 64, 70*f*
Glassarian fissures 5
Glomus
  jugulare 74
  tumors 73
  tympanicum 73, 73*f*
Glossopharyngeal nerve 9, 25
Greater superficial petrosal nerve 48, 48*f*, 51
Gusher syndrome 51

H

Hairs, absence of 14
Hamulus 58*f*
Hemifacial spasm 51
Henle's spine 6*f*, 37
High-resolution computed tomography 67, 70*f*
  temporal bone 44*f*
His hillock 11
Human skull, development of 2*f*
Hyperintense 62
Hypotympanic fissure 16
Hypotympanum 25, 26

I

Incudal fold
  posterior 34
  superior 33, 34*f*
Incudomalleal fold, lateral 34

Incus 23, 23*f*
  short process of 53
Inferior tympanic artery 62*f*
Infralabyrinthine 42*f*
  cell 40
Internal auditory canal 7, 40, 45, 70*f*
Internal auditory meatus 6*f*, 47*f*, 50, 63, 67*f*
  upper part of 64*f*
Internal carotid artery 15, 17*f*, 52*f*, 58*f*, 70*f*
Internal petrosquamous fissure 5
Intracranial segment 45
Isthmus 56
Iter chordae
  anterior 18
  posterior 18

J

Jacobson's nerve 25
Jacobson's preganglionic fibers 25
Jugular bulb 17, 17*f*, 66*f*, 67, 68*f*
  dehiscent 17
  enlarged 74
  high 17, 17*f*
Jugular foramen 63
Jugular fossa 7*f*, 68

K

Keratosis obturans 73
Korner's septum 5, 9, 13*f*, 31, 31*f*, 32*f*, 38, 38*f*

L

Labyrinthine
  artery 51
  segment 45, 50
Labyrinthitis 71
  chronic 71
Lacrimatory nucleus 45
Lamina propria 18
Laryngopharyngeal reflux 59
Levator veli palatini 57
  muscle 58*f*
Longitudinal fracture 71
  transverse fracture 71

M

MacEwen triangle 9, 37
Magnetic resonance imaging 61, 62, 74, 74*f*

Malformations, congenital 69
Malleal ligament, anterior 23, 32
Malleolal fold, superior 33, 34*f*
Malleus 23*f*, 49*f*
  head of 70*f*
  lateral process of 18*f*
Mandibular fossa 8*f*
Mastoid 21*f*, 35, 40, 67, 71*f*
  air cell 36*f*
    system 39, 39*fc*
  antrum 37, 64*f*
    deep relations of 37*f*
  artery 25
  bone 8, 8*f*
  cavity 41*f*
  development of 13
  pneumatization 40*f*, 41*f*
    degree of 40*f*
  process 53
  segment 45, 67*f*
  tip 53
McEwen's triangle 8
Meatal segment 45
Medial saccule 30
Meningioma 73
Meningocele 71
Meningoencephalocele 71
Mesotympanum 22*f*, 25
Middle ear 27*f*
  blood vessels 25
  cavity 11, 15*f*, 22*f*
    superior wall of 16*f*
  cleft 13
  compartments of 25*f*, 30
  folds 33*f*
  muscles 24
  ossicles 22*f*
  spaces, embryology of 12*fc*, 13*f*, 31*f*, 31*fc*
  structures 48*f*
  surgical floor of 19
Middle meningeal artery, branch of 51
Modiolus lamina 69
Muscles 57

N

Nasopharynx 56, 57*f*
  tumors 59
Nervus intermedius 47
Neuritis 72
Neuroma 73

O

Obstruction, anatomical 59
Ossicles 19*f*, 65*f*
Ossicular chain 22
    development of 12
Ostmann's pad 57, 57*f*, 59
Otic capsule 3*f*, 70*f*
    cartilaginous 45
Otitis media, acute 59*f*
Otodystrophies 74
Otomastoiditis
    acute 71
    chronic 71, 72*f*
Otorrhea 51
Otosclerosis 23, 74, 75
Outer attic wall 19*f*
    computed tomography image of 19*f*

P

Paratubal muscles 58*f*
Parotid 51*f*
    gland 49
        surgery 53
Pars
    flaccida 18*f*
    nervosa, posterior 5
    tensa 18, 26*f*
    venosa, anterior 5
Perifacial cell 42*f*
Perifenestral otosclerosis 21
Perilabyrinthine cell 40
    tracts 42*f*
Petromastoid cell 9
Petrosal artery, superior 51
Petrosquamous fissures 5
Petrotympanic fissure 5, 6*f*, 18
Petrous apex 6*f*, 40, 69
    cholesteatoma of 73, 73*f*
Petrous bone 5
    anterior surface of 6*f*
    posterior face of 6*f*
Pharyngobasilar fascia 56
Pneumatization
    degree of 40*fc*
    tract of 36*fc*
Postauricular artery, branch of 51
Posterior fossa dural plate 38
Posteromedial tract 40
Processus cochleariformis 53
Protein-rich mucus 62
Protympanum 25, 26

Prussak's space 18, 19, 19*f*, 30, 35, 63
    anterior limit of 32
    isolated 26*f*
    roof of 32
Pyramidal eminence 21, 22, 24*f*, 45, 65*f*

R

Ramsay-Hunt syndrome 72
Reichert's cartilage 11, 14
Retrofacial air cells 26
Retrofacial dissection 41
Retrotympanum 25, 26
Rivinus notch 12*f*, 18
Round window niche 65, 66*f*

S

Saccule 24*f*
    anterior 30
    posterior 30
Saccus
    anticus 12, 30
    medius 30
    posticus 30, 31
    superior 30
Salivatory nucleus, superior 45
Salpingopharyngeus 57
Schwann cells, multiple 49
Sclerotic mastoid 40*f*
Scutum 7*f*, 18
    erosion 63
Semicircular canal
    horizontal 53
    lateral 20, 40*f*, 48, 48*f*, 52*f*, 53, 63
    posterior 37
Sensorineural deafness 70
Shrapnell's membrane 18
Sigmoid sinus 38
Sinodural angle 38
    cadaveric picture of 39*f*
Sinus morgagni 56
Sinus tympani 27, 27*f*, 63
    small 28
    types of 28
Skull
    coronal section of 4*f*
    infant 4*f*
Spiral lamina 69
Stapedial artery 44
Stapedius muscle 24*f*
Stapes 23

Styloid
    apparatus 8
    bone 8*f*
    eminences 22
    process 1, 6*f*-8*f*, 53
Stylomastoid
    artery 25, 51, 52*f*
    foramen 4*f*, 7*f*, 45, 48
Subarachnoid space 15
Subarcuate fossa 9
Subarcuate tract 41
Sulcus tubae 56
Superficial petrosal artery 25, 52*f*
Superior semicircular canal 21*f*, 37, 63, 63*f*, 64*f*
    prominence of 6
Supralabyrinthine 42*f*
    cell 40
Supratubal recess 26, 26*f*, 52*f*

T

Tegmen 68
    plate 14
    tympani 14, 15, 25
        preservation of 15
Temporal artery, middle 8*f*
Temporal bone 1, 1*f*, 6*f*, 11, 67, 70*f*
    computed tomography scan of 9
    congenital anomalies of 69
    development of 1
    inferior surface of 7*f*
    lateral surface of 8*f*
    petrous part of 5*f*
    pneumatisation 41*f*
    radiology of 61, 61*f*
    squamous part of 8*f*
    superior surface of 64*f*
    surface anatomy of 5
    trauma 71
    tympanic part of 7*f*
Temporomandibular joint 57*f*
Tensor tympani 57
    fold 34, 34*f*
    muscle 24*f*, 52*f*
Tensor veli palatini 57, 58*f*
Tractus solitaries, nucleus of 45
Tragal cartilage pointer 53
Trautmann's triangle 39
Tubal
    artery 25
    cartilage 58*f*
    fibrous membrane 58*f*
    ligament 58*f*
    lumen 58*f*

Tubotympanic recess 3*f*, 12*fc*
Tumor 62
Tympani orifice 56
Tympanic artery
    anterior 25, 52*f*
    superior 52*f*
Tympanic bone 7, 12*f*, 26
    abnormal development of 51
Tympanic cavity 14, 17*f*, 50
    anterior wall of 21
    floor of 15
    lateral wall of 17
    medial wall of 19
    nerves of 25
    posterior wall of 21
    roof of 14
Tympanic diaphragm 30
Tympanic isthmus 30, 35
Tympanic membrane 18, 33*f*
    normal 18*f*
Tympanic plexus 58
Tympanic ring 7*f*
Tympanic segment 45, 48, 49*f*
Tympanic sinus, lateral 27
Tympanic spine 18
    anterior 12*f*
    posterior 12*f*
Tympanomalleal fold
    anterior 32
    posterior 32
Tympanomastoid compartment 13
    development of 11
    surgical anatomy of 30
Tympanomastoid fissure 6*f*
Tympanomastoid surgeries 15
Tympanomastoid suture 14, 53
Tympanosquamous fissure 7*f*
Tympanosquamous suture 6*f*, 14
Tympanotomy, posterior 21

U

Utricle 24*f*

V

Vascular strips 14
Vertical facial nerve 27*f*
Vertigo 71
Vestibular duct 6*f*
Vestibular nerve, superior 64*f*
Vestibular schwannoma 74, 74*f*
Vestibule 65*f*, 67*f*
von Troeltsch
    anterior pouch 12, 26*f*, 32
    posterior pouch 19, 26, 26*f*

W

Watery mucus 62

Z

Zygomatic arch 25
Zygomatic process 8. 8*f*

EU GSPR Authorised Reprsentative
Logos Europe, 9 rue Nicolas Poussin
1700, La Rochelle, France
Phone: +33 (0) 6 67 93 73 78
E-mail: contact@logoseurope.eu

www.ingramcontent.com/pod-product-compliance
Ingram Content Group UK Ltd.
Pitfield, Milton Keynes, MK11 3LW, UK
UKHW051559010326

468476UK00022B/16